Queer Psychoanalysis

Queer Psychoanalysis offers a detailed study of the tensions and contiguities between the field of queer theory and that of Freudian-Lacanian metapsychology.

Drawing on a detailed reading of the critiques that have been levelled against psychoanalysis by queer theorists, this book makes use of, and reinvigorates, a certain ethics. Fabrice Bourlez offers a perspective from which these two domains, rather than being opposed one to the other, can be thought of as being in dialogue. The book considers the work of both queer theorists and psychoanalytic thinkers and confronts the numerous homophobic stances that punctuate the history of psychanalysis. Bourlez formulates a manner of thinking that frees psychoanalysis from its preconceptions and unthought, while avoiding the entrapment of queer theory in a self-righteous utopian ideal. In so doing, this book conceptualizes a vision of psychanalysis that is better able to attend to the full spectrum of contemporary subjects.

Queer Psychoanalysis will be essential reading for psychoanalysts and for scholars of psychoanalytic studies, sexuality, gender studies, psychology, cultural studies, aesthetic studies, and queer theory.

Fabrice Bourlez is a psychoanalyst based in Paris, France. He also teaches aesthetics at ESAD in Reims and is co-holder of the Chair of Troubles, Alliances, and Aesthetics at ENSBA in Paris.

The Lines of the Symbolic in Psychoanalysis Series

Series Editor: Ian Parker, Manchester Psychoanalytic Matrix

Psychoanalytic clinical and theoretical work is always embedded in specific linguistic and cultural contexts and carries their traces, traces which this series attends to in its focus on multiple contradictory and antagonistic 'lines of the Symbolic'. This series takes its cue from Lacan's psychoanalytic work on three registers of human experience, the Symbolic, the Imaginary and the Real, and employs this distinctive understanding of cultural, communication and embodiment to link with other traditions of cultural, clinical and theoretical practice beyond the Lacanian symbolic universe. The Lines of the Symbolic in Psychoanalysis Series provides a reflexive reworking of theoretical and practical issues, translating psychoanalytic writing from different contexts, grounding that work in the specific histories and politics that provide the conditions of possibility for its descriptions and interventions to function. The series makes connections between different cultural and disciplinary sites in which psychoanalysis operates, questioning the idea that there could be one single correct reading and application of Lacan. Its authors trace their own path, their own line through the Symbolic, situating psychoanalysis in relation to debates which intersect with Lacanian work, explicating it, extending it and challenging it.

Decolonization and Psychoanalysis
The Underside of Signification
Ahmad Fuad Rahmat

Queer Theory, Lacanian Psychoanalysis, Sexual Politics
From Norm to Desire
Luiz Valle Junior

Taking Back Desire
A Psychoanalytic Approach to Queerness and Neoliberalism on Screen
James Lawrence Slattery

On the Theory and Clinic of Lacanian Psychoanalysis: Speaking of Lacan
Chris Vanderwees

Queer Psychoanalysis: Minor Clinic and Deconstruction of Gender
Fabrice Bourlez

For more information about the series, please visit: https://www.routledge.com/The-Lines-of-the-Symbolic-in-Psychoanalysis-Series/book-series/KARNLOS

Queer Psychoanalysis

Minor Clinic and Deconstruction of Gender

Fabrice Bourlez

Routledge
Taylor & Francis Group
LONDON AND NEW YORK

First published 2026
by Routledge
4 Park Square, Milton Park, Abingdon, Oxon OX14 4RN

and by Routledge
605 Third Avenue, New York, NY 10158

Routledge is an imprint of the Taylor & Francis Group, an informa business

Designed cover image: Laura Bottereau & Marine Fiquet, Morceaux synthétiques, © Adagp, Paris, 2022.

Translated from the French, *Queer psychanalyse* © 2018, HERMANN, www.editions-hermann.fr

British Library Cataloguing in Publication Data
A catalogue record for this book is available from the British Library

ISBN: 9781041010302 (hbk)
ISBN: 9781041010296 (pbk)
ISBN: 9781003612735 (ebk)

DOI: 10.4324/9781003612735

Typeset in Times New Roman
by Taylor & Francis Books

Contents

Contents

Series preface for Fabrice Bourlez's *Queer Psychoanalysis*

Psychoanalysis has always been queer, disturbing taken-for-granted binary categories of sex and gender, opening a place in the clinic for the subject to question what they have been told they are as a man or a woman as well as who they should think they are as a good boy or good girl. Psychoanalysis, in its fidelity to the founding texts of Freud and Lacan and many others, has also always opened itself to new readings, re-readings, twisted returns, that show the intrinsic ambiguity that hides inside each and every apparently definite statement about what constitutes human subjectivity.

This ambiguity bears on the stories told about Oedipus, for instance, and the place of Oedipus in myth, medicine and then in the travails of the Symbolic order, including what strange detours each and every subject takes through the heteronormative straits of what is usually taken to be their 'development'. One of the traps that many ostensibly subversive readings of key psychoanalytic texts risk falling into is that the restrictive adaptive modes of explanation in heteronormative psychoanalysis are, at one moment, refused, but then to be replaced with yet another account that universalises and essentialises subjectivity.

This book carefully and cleverly skirts around that kind of trap, showing us that inside the apparently prescriptive accounts of sex and gender that lace together the peculiar symbolic order that is psychoanalytic discourse, there are multiple competing descriptions that offer a more generous open account of what a human subject might be. It is not necessary to 'imaginarise' elements of the symbolic in order to forge an identity, and queer psychoanalysis, indeed, avoids replacing the straight lines of the symbolic with the lures of an identitarian imaginary.

Time and again, claims are made in psychoanalysis about what the bedrock of human experience is, sometimes appealing to biology, sometimes appealing to societal strictures. But a queer re-reading of psychoanalysis shows us that, just as surely as we can open up the symbolic order to different readings, just as surely as we can steer clear of an imaginary image of ourselves that the symbolic structures for us, so we can find a way to encounter the real, not as brute nature but as a meshwork of contradictions.

Those contradictions, themselves, are the conceptual basis of queer psychoanalysis.

Psychoanalytic clinical and theoretical work circulates through multiple intersecting antagonistic symbolic universes. This series opens connections between different cultural sites in which Lacanian work has developed in distinctive ways, in forms of work that question the idea that there could be any single correct reading and application. The Lines of the Symbolic in Psychoanalysis series provides a reflexive reworking of psychoanalysis that transmits Lacanian writing from around the world, steering a course between the temptations of a metalanguage and imaginary reduction, between the claim to provide a god's eye view of psychoanalysis and the idea that psychoanalysis must everywhere be the same. And the elaboration of psychoanalysis in the symbolic here grounds its theory and practice in the history and politics of the work in a variety of interventions that touch the real.

Ian Parker
Manchester Psychoanalytic Matrix

Chapter 1

Undoing Analysis

Writing

I am writing for my friends. My homosexual friends, both men and women, gay, lesbian, bisexual, trans, and *queer*... all of those who have crossed the threshold of a psychoanalytic practice and who have chosen not to stay. I am writing for those who have read works critical of psychoanalysis, and who have found truth in these brilliant, acerbic, harsh, and astute texts, raging against the psychoanalytic field. I am writing for those who have been left angered by their encounter with the unconscious. And for those who refuse to read Freud on principle, and who believe, with faith set in stone, that Lacan was a mere phallogocentric homophobe.

I am writing for my philosopher friends, so often convinced of the lack of depth in the work published in the wake of gay and lesbian studies, of queer theory, and of trans and porn studies. As well as for those who yearn for rigour and decency, who appeal as much to biological clarity, and to the reality of the body, as to the immutability of the natural order, the Universal, and Reason. Often, these are the same friends who laugh at the long years that they have spent on the analytical couch shelling out their suffering. Neither free associative flights of fancy, nor associatory communitarianism meet with their favour. For them, true reflection should be distrustful of indiscriminate verbiage, of academic digressions, and of linguistic divulgations. They wish to remain grounded, and cling to a vision of reality founded on a single, shared world, guided by enlightenment, rigour, and clarity, as well as by unity and ordered thinking.

I am writing for my friends, psychoanalysts, who labour patiently in the shadows and who, in their practice, encounter both the quotidian and more profound woes of their patients. More or less sheltered, and most often ensconced in an enigmatic silence, day after day, they find the strength to reflect upon the unique nature of their role, which is to listen. They wish to defend the specificity of strange encounters, where contemporary life is woven from snippets, segments, and fragmented stories. Encounters where the most vivid aspects of both the immutable and the mutable are brought

DOI: 10.4324/9781003612735-1

forth. Convinced of the significance of their practice, they forever seek to reveal the value of the atypical, the inopportune, and the merits of psychoanalysis for one and for all. Taking up such a daring challenge occasionally means that it is necessary to abandon the habitual prudence of the analytic field and its semantic, meta-psychological, and clinical cues in order to affirm without ambiguity, and stake out a clear position. This implies taking a step *Outside*, [1] taking in the zeitgeist, the desideratum of the marginalized and of minorities, and, without retreating in the face of ideological, social, and political pressures, continue to reinvest themselves in their toil.

I am writing with all my heart, from my position as a homosexual, as a psychoanalyst, as a desiring subject. I am convinced of the necessity of this book, which, no doubt, may occasionally seem more like a call to action than a reasoned line of thought. I have, no doubt, failed to extinguish the fires of activism that burn within. And I could, no doubt, foreground the performative aspect of this book in lieu of its argumentation. But in the perimeter defined by the analytic space, as in that which is defined by homosexuality, is it not always necessary to break the silence, especially when the latter is a synonym of repression? Is it not forever necessary to break down any resistance, and to thus allow for the free expression of desire?

Resisting

Psychoanalysis is a unique experience. It lightens the load of being. It opens one to joy and to becoming. The following pages aim to reinvent the words for that which can be said (*le dire*): by reconsidering texts which excoriate psychoanalytic theory, I would like to continue to enliven psychoanalytic praxis. In this, it is necessary to distinguish the siren song and polemical fires of the present, to take note of what has changed, and what continues unceasingly to evolve in terms of gender and sexuality, in terms of our way of life, our suffering, and the manner in which we love. In order to be receptive, both through speech and through the act of listening, to the torments of one and of all, it seemed useful to me to dare appropriate the discourse and the concepts, the critiques and the precepts, which are alien or opposed to those whose practice is predicated upon the hypothesis of the unconscious. Both sides have landed fierce blows to the sound of reverberating battle cries. Yet this strategy does not so much seek to dodge or minimize these criticisms, than to reappropriate their strength and anger, and put them to work in awakening desire.

From the moment of its emergence on the intellectual scene, psychoanalysis has been the subject of an ever-increasing list of grievances. This is, however, not to say that one should abandon psychoanalysis as a clinical practice, nor put an end to the vagaries[2] that prevail along the pathway to the cure. Indeed, for Freud, criticism represented a form of resistance to his breakthrough. His argument is, essentially, irrefutable: "the truth that I have set forth is of such a magnitude, that it may seem unbearable to you." But this has never been a sufficiently valid excuse to let sleeping dogs lie. Both Freud and Lacan, as well as all their true heirs, are called upon to defend the specificity of the psychoanalytic approach, to modestly attempt to carry forth the torch, to continue the work of comprehending the incomprehensible, of understanding that which renders incomparable the narrative of our lives.

Change is always associated with that which comes from the Outside, that which erupts upon the psychoanalytic scene in a contrary movement, embodied in ideological, philosophical, and partisan deconstructions. This exteriority inserts itself into our practice and bades us not submit. We are bidden to neither reiterate nor to systematize. In short, we are commanded to create. The controversies surrounding femininities, masculinities, motherhood, fatherhood, and parenthood appear to no longer be blatantly clear but form part of a constellation of concepts which are defined in relation to a given point in time. They change, they shift, they are overturned, they are unsettled, nothing is as it was before. The demands of "postfeminism," as articulated in gender and queer studies, have by and large contributed to the weakening of all connections between the real and the natural.

The most well-known exponents of gender studies have themselves insisted upon the necessity of understanding the plurality of the methods and structures that they seek to develop.[3] This plurality can be found in the manner in which these theories seek to extend the possibilities of existence. The sum total of their ideas aims at extending the scope of what can be seen as enviable modes of living. To this end, numerous theoreticians, whose studies focus on the question of gender, wish to unpick the tapestry of norms, cutting apart the moral constraints which stigmatize or marginalize certain forms of sexual orientation, certain types of relationship, or certain forms of kinship. This foregrounds an inclusive, as opposed to an exclusive, mode of thought. These theories have, thus, slowly but surely, and in an almost ideological manner, offered a glimmer of hope to some, while for others they represent the multi-headed Hydra. For the latter, gender studies itself, and all that it represents, should be expeditiously dispatched, lest civilization itself be irrevocably plunged into crisis.

In this context, psychoanalysis can be considered to be the guarantor of the symbolic order: a respected doctrine that is able to offer stable landmarks to the directionless. The most militant gender theorists have nevertheless insisted upon the static nature of psychoanalysis. And the *queer* movement itself has risen up against psychoanalysis, illustrating the manner in which, as opposed to supporting change, the conceptual apparatus of psychoanalysis tends to condemn it. One should, moreover, recognize that the positions which have been staked out by a number of students of the unconscious have contributed to the entrenchment of psychoanalysis as a normative instance, capable of stigmatizing, judging, and opposing the recognition of certain forms of love, kinship, parenthood, and bodies in so far as they do not conform, are considered deviant, or simply in so far as they exist too far outside the Freudian order of things. Gays, lesbians, trans, bi, queers, feminists – those who we can succinctly consider in Deleuzian terms, as belonging to the Minority: that is to say those who exist on the margins of society, and those who, explicitly, do not conform to the white heterosexual form of kinship, those who are in the Minority not in mere numerical terms, but in terms of their access to power and the ability to express themselves and their truth publicly – have often lamented the aforementioned positions. They bemoan the stigmatization to which they have been victim as a result of convictions grounded in theory, and as a result of the attitude of certain analysts who, in reinforcing those convictions, have caused substantial harm.

The insistence with which these wounds have been brandished as a weapon against psychoanalysis in particular, and against the psychological field of study in general, cannot be simply brushed aside in an unspecified appeal to the laws of the unconscious, or to a deeper investigation lacking any concrete impact. My hypothesis is simple. While these critiques can perhaps be seen to attest to a degree of resistance regarding the analytical cause, this does not necessarily invalidate their general scope. Rather, they can be seen to illuminate a way Outside, charting a new path for psychoanalysts who have become overly enmeshed in the boundaries of their practice, concentrating too long upon the "inexistence of the sexual relation" at the risk of disavowing that which, indeed, does exist. Our goal is to (re)dress these wounds.

Coming out

It thus seemed inevitable to me, not so much as to convince, but to express, to reiterate, to explain. And this, beginning with that which unmistakably, like it or not, colours my activities. Here we have it. Call me "gay." Proclaim that I am "bent." Refer to me as a "fag." Malign me as a "fairy." Take me under your protective and understanding wing. Or would you prefer to know nothing of this? Turn a deaf ear. It matters little to me. I have said it.

This is a preliminary declaration: a starting point from which we can *figure out* a *gay science*. Neither communitarian, nor assimilationist, I have understood that, whether it be upon, or behind the analytic couch, to speak is to awaken desire. Thus, for a long time, I have chosen to speak of *this*, to take *this* on, to reclaim my right to consider *this* less as a banner than as a laboratory. A homosexuality unmarked by psychological depth and by diagnostic pathologization. Rather, this would form a prism for thoughtful reflection, or a means for the translation of discourse: a mirror, if you will, where narcissism is erased and from which a single piercing gaze emerges, that of a difference capable of sowing turmoil in the thoughts we take for granted.

Setting the context of a given thought implies removing the veneer of objectivity, showing the degree to which appeals to neutrality, to sacrosanct transparency, and to an all-powerful Universalism, merely disguise existing power relations. In too often seeking to describe things in a positivist manner, we end up thinking that they are as they are, because that is how they *should* be: we forget to interrogate alternative ways of envisioning the world. To consider the origin of a statement, is, to my mind, to highlight that to which we are opposed.

And yet, why begin with such an extravagant declaration? Why, devil-may-care, expose one's private life at the very onset? Is the analyst's first task not that of measured silence? By beginning on such a personal note, laying bare this intimate distinctiveness, this particular feeling, are we not deprived of all argumentative rigour? Does this not skew our reasoning from the very start?

It seems to me that the singularity of my desire is not easily divorced from my sexual orientation. This, perhaps, gives me an advantage in understanding and lending an ear to stigmatization, discrimination, and hatred. Indeed, my personal experience of the psychoanalytic cure has convinced me of the importance of finding the root cause of one's desire so as to succeed in moving forward in both a public and in a private sense.

Therefore, and please allow me to insist on this point: what happens when "crazy" is confronted by "queer" in an analytic space? Is the queer condemned to the couch? Will the queer be told that he is taking up too much space, and that he needs to de-pathologize himself before attempting to treat others? And yet, does a clinical encounter not accept a degree of incurability? Who is truly ill in this encounter? He who tells the queer to return to his cage,[4] or the madman who takes on the responsibility of treating the queer? Unless it is, quite simply, he who designates mad from mad and queer from queer – the guarantor of norms.

Coming out of the closet is a first step, and we have now left our naughty little secret behind. We have acknowledged a part of who we are. It is a gesture, a trope, a performance. Today still, knowing or not knowing, saying these words or leaving them unsaid, still implies new power relations. To this end it is better to be clear from the outset: this is not an exercise in which the minority card is played within the psychoanalytic session, to prove one's credentials, to say "I am one of you, I understand." This is not where the stakes lie, and I have never had any intention of revealing even the slightest aspect of my private life to a patient. On the contrary, to confirm from the very beginning, in a book that lies in the space between theory and clinical practice, that one is both a homosexual *and* a psychoanalyst offers an opportunity to take a fresh look at the consequences of this declaration. These consequences are at once of the institutional, political, and the ethical order. In writing, and in thinking through this double specificity without shame or embarrassment, one can envision the field of militant ideologies, and that of psychoanalysis, along more innovative paths. Tackling analytic theory from an uncommon angle is, as always, to follow one's desire, but in this case, it is to follow a desire that arises out of one's affiliation to a minority. So be it: I am a shrink and a faggot. I've said it, I've repeated it, and I'll return to it. Better get used to it.

Queer psychoanalysis

The oddness of this preamble is of particular proximity to the consonance of my title: "*queer* psychoanalysis." Indeed, how is one to understand this title? In the beginning, in English, the word *queer* meant bizarre or strange, later becoming an insult that was used to denigrate homosexuals in the same vein as faggot, or pansy. Over the last 30 years however, *queer* has become a militant rallying cry: "In so far as you call us perverts, faggots, pansies, strange and unnatural, understand that we are! Understand too that this state of affairs will probably persist!" This self-same rallying cry cleared the way not only for an incalculable number of political demonstrations, but also for numerous novel theoretical considerations. The word *queer* is abuzz with thoughts and actions which advocate for the lives of unruly and edgy bodies, bodies motivated by desires and of an appearance that some may find disturbing. These thoughts and these actions, these bodies, and these lives seek to affirm themselves in their exceptional banality.

We could thus say that "queer psychoanalysis" is a "psychoanalysis of the faggot" –although the humorousness of this expression would seem to preclude the necessary gravitas. Yet, if we were to listen more carefully, queer psychoanalysis resonates in an alternate manner. That is to say that the signifying ambiguity contained within this expression echoes what we can interpret as a question regarding psychoanalytic praxis itself. Qu'*ear* psychoanalysis? To what does psychoanalysis lend its ear? What do psychoanalysts hear with their ear to the ground? What are we even to understand by psychoanalysis today? Hear ye, hear ye, queer theory questions the scope of your silence, and of your well-meaning, evenly suspended attention.

Unless one is to understand this expression less as a question, than as an affirmation: queer psychoanalysis. Freudian practice, even before the advent of sexual liberation, was resolutely concerned with the bizarre and the strange, drawn to a non-biological polymorphous perversion. Listen up you angry minorities, that which you castigate with such dogged determination, participates in – and even anticipates – the development and revolution of the field of sexualities. What is more, without psychoanalysis your outcries would have wound up as whispers. There is a kernel of queer in psychoanalysis itself, in the disturbing, the strange, the unruly, the prideful. Free association, dreams, the way in which our bodies experience ecstasy, even the drives, all contain an element of queer.

So how should one hear queer? What do queer peoples, those who deconstruct gender and norms, understand when it comes to the unsettling uncanniness of psychoanalysis?

These questions are voluntarily provocative. They call into question both theory and practice. They point out the political implications of psychoanalysis, and the effect that it has on reality itself. To this end, it is worth noting from the get-go, that both psychoanalysis and queer shuffle back and forth between theory and practice. No psychoanalysis without a clinic, no analyst without an act, no queer theory without action, no queers without a struggle. In each of these examples, understanding is built out of experience. Out with armchair theorization, any conceptual house of cards, or overly abstract argumentation. We think, we write, and we read in order to do better when faced with the unbearable, subverting the ways in which we live, love, and intellectualize.

So, given this proximity, could we undertake a task of cultural translation between some critical concepts that lie on the margins of queer theory, and some that form part of psychoanalytic ethics? How should the grievances of those who feel that they are victims of systemic (economic, political, social, identitarian…) oppression be heeded? How to avoid the tactlessness of such systems of oppression within the context of the psychoanalytic cure? How, as an analyst, can one sidestep becoming a mere cog in the wheel? How can one chart a concrete path forward, which enables one to reconsider the formulations by which the psychoanalytic clinic is orientated, without too quickly taking them for granted? Can we, without balking at the effort, demonstrate the utility of renewing the acuity and the rigour of psychoanalysis, not so much for all as for every *one*? In so doing, what queer does for psychoanalysis, psychoanalysis pays back in return.

To this end, and some time ago already, activist and queer philosopher Paul Beatriz Preciado threw down a gauntlet which has, it seems to me, remained unanswered. In a text that lies half-way between theory and fiction, Preciado offers a breathtaking narration, perhaps even a tribute, to gender rebellion, to *hacking* the body itself. For Preciado the body is not natural, in and of itself, and, in so far as it is not natural: why not construct another? Why does one have to submit oneself to the binary gender assignment of male/female? Why not voluntarily hack oneself, in the same way that others hack IT or banking systems? At the time, the philosopher who today identifies as male, self-administered testosterone using patches in an analogous manner to a junkie shooting up intravenously. Over a period of nine months, Preciado described the bodily effects of this hormonal modification.

To a greater and greater degree, techno-digital prosthetics ensnare our bodies in a caress, and to a greater and greater degree the natural is erased in favour of the artificial. Bodies in the pharmaco-pornographic society move forward as subjectivities ensnared by norms, apparatuses, constructions, and configurations. These are at once symbolic, concrete, and virtual. From before our birth, until the moment of our death, technology has engulfed our very existence,[5] setting the tempo. Such an understanding of subjectivity draws on the heritage of Michel Foucault, and in particular on the notion of biopower. We can understand biopower as that which, instead of manifesting itself through the limitation of freedoms, through the right of death, or through a clearly identified law, now is manifest in the expression of a constant yet vague control over our lives. This control takes the form of the production of norms which, taking hold of our very bodies, and exerting a degree of control over them, encourage certain forms of enjoyment or ecstasy to the exclusion of others. In such a society, gender constructions are not only simple processes of linguistic categorization, but also material processes through which the body itself is constructed (corset, speculum, vibrator, dildo, webcam…).[6]

Should such radical change reduce us to tears? Should we dig in our heels and insist on the limited scope echoed in this line of reasoning? Does psychoanalysis, as a practice, not offer a counterbalance to such encouragements towards self-metamorphosis? And, on the contrary, have these changes not had any impact on the knowledge gleaned from the unconscious? Should we remain stoic? Neither one, nor the other. In taking these observations as his starting point, Preciado extends an invitation, aspiring to a *queeranalysis*:

> *Queeranalysis* isn't against psychoanalysis, but it goes beyond it by politicizing it […]. *Queeranalysis* is a practice that, instead of conceptualizing gender and sexual dissent through a lens of psychological pathology […], would conceive of normalization and its effects as biopolitical […]. *Queeranalysis* does not reject […] the analysis of dreams, the talking cure, hypnosis […] but it attacks […] the rhetoric of gender, sex, race, disability, and class at work in these psychotherapeutic practices.[7]

Here, it is no longer a question of fighting *against* psychoanalysis. Rather, the idea is to take on a new challenge: to show that the relationship between gender de-construction and psychoanalysis is not so much one of opposition than of an embrace. *Against* but not *opposed*: intertwined.

A clinic in a minor key

Of course, psychoanalysis doesn't exist as a singular, unified theoretical domain. There are only psychoanalysts, that is to say practitioners of various approaches, including those who authorise *themselves*, who engage in analysis, and who practice in the aforementioned domain. In order to garner a better view of this nebulous domain, this infinite constellation of opposed and complementary *modus operandi*, allow me to propose that psychoanalysis and analytically orientated therapies, therapeutic assessment, or the clinical encounter can be articulated in two manners, that is, in two modes that we could refer to as a clinic "in a major key" and as a clinic "in a minor key."[8]

This distinction is drawn from the work of Gilles Deleuze and Félix Guattari on the language of literature. By "major" the authors envisage a certain manner of using language which fixes linguistic variables in place, so as to establish a constant. This allows for the particular circumstances of a given articulation to be glossed over, ensuring its transcendental and sovereign regulation, which in turn prescribes the logic of expression. Employing a language in a "major" mode, in so far as it remains foreign to the inherent variations of each given situation, imposes itself as an act of domination, as a universally self-evident reference point. In a "major" mode, language is recognizable, understandable, and relatable: it's Victor Hugo's use of French, or Goethe's use of German, and, without a doubt, Aristotle's use of Greek.

> How many people today live in a language that is not their own? Or no longer, or not yet, even know their own and know poorly the major language that they are forced to serve? This is the problem of immigrants, and especially of their children, the problem of minorities, the problem of a minor literature, but also a problem for all of us: how to tear a minor literature away from its own language, allowing it to challenge the language and making it follow a sober revolutionary path? How to become a nomad and an immigrant and a gypsy in relation to one's own language?[9]

All literature that seeks to change the modes of perception and of expression has a responsibility to be seen as a minor literature.

Major literature is characteristically inscribed within tradition and conservation, being articulated through the defence of a pre-existing status quo. On the contrary, the use of minor literature is a revolutionary step in relation to language itself: lending new intensities and novel reverberations to that which it effectively deterritorialises. Approaching language from the position of a minor literature is to tie the language and the tongue, the utterance and the subject to political issues. For Deleuze and Guattari, "a rule of grammar is a power marker before it is a syntactical marker."[10] And, further on: "forming grammatically correct sentences is for the normal individual the prerequisite for any submission to social laws. No one is supposed to be ignorant of grammaticality; those who are belong in special institutions. The unity of language is fundamentally political."[11]

The use of minor literature plugs the individual and their modes of expression into something other than themselves. It liberates existence from the prison of grammar, propelling it beyond preestablished meanings. It undermines what has been taken for granted and what follows is a near mathematical process of reduction, of becoming minor. From shifts in meaning, from statements and formulas, we subtract their connection to the personal and the psychological. Stability is set aside, and what emerges is polyphonic, open and multiple: a series of connections that are no longer symbolic but micropolitical. By breaking through the certainties of what constitutes speaking, "language stops being representative in order to now move toward its extremities or its limits."[12]

Minor literature seeks to draw near to the infinite variations implied by a given linguistic layout. Its Kafka's German, Beckett's French, and Pasolini's Italian: foreign languages within their own language, to paraphrase the well-known Proustian formulation, defying the dictates of grammar and of the mother tongue. That which is constant is replaced by continuous variation: "Placing elements of any nature in continuous variation is an operation that will perhaps give rise to new distinctions, but takes none as final and has none in advance."[13] Through their use of language in a minor mode, those who are habitually sworn to silence are able to reappropriate the expressive domain. They unlock the effervescence of language and its rules as the hitherto unthinkable is drawn forth. They disentangle themselves from language in a "major mode," and this strange "taste for dominants, constants, and universals."[14] They propel that which seems as though it should be, for all time and eternity, into a "specific, unforeseen, autonomous becoming."[15]

Drawing on this distinction, we could envisage two features, two customs, two manners of relating to psychoanalysis. A clinic in a major key would offer *the* veritable form of theoretic conservatism. After nearly a century, Lady Psychoanalysis, draped in her mysterious silence, is quick to be the judge of good morals and conduct. Steeped in respectability, she condemns with supreme condescending confidence and differential diagnoses the affairs of the heart, the ways of life, and the forms of sexuality that do not measure up to her benchmark.

It is to this major mode, in both clinical practice and scientific literature, that the gender de-constructionists are opposed, in both their publications and in their work more generally. Reading the critiques levelled by Deleuze and Guattari,[16] to begin with, often leaves clinicians feeling ill at ease. Faced with these politico-theoretical criticisms, a sense of injustice rears its head. Does the analyst not spend his time in silence so as to allow the subject to "pronounce before him the very words in which he recognizes the law of his own being"[17]? Does he who has devoted his life in order to "ignore what he knows,"[18] have no other choice than to practise psychoanalysis in a minor mode? Without a doubt. In this case, the vicious vituperations of Deleuze and Guattari, like those of the queer, merit a fresh reminder of what Freud and Lacan have already insisted upon:

> For psychoanalysis is also a practice subordinated by its purpose to what is most particular about the subject. And when Freud emphasizes this, going so far as to say that the analytic science must be called back into question in the analysis of each case [...] he quite clearly indicates to the analysand the path his training should follow.[19]

Nearly 40 years later, for Deleuze and Guattari, as for Preciado, the call to criticism and to liberation passes through the unconscious. To avoid being merely reactionary, it is necessary to unceasingly question the manner in which we address the unconscious. To be precise, to practice psychoanalysis in a minor mode would be tantamount to identifying the spaces where the analytic exercise echoes in non-conformity, and to play upon the breaking points in the psychoanalytic doxa. In short, this would be to question that which, for psychoanalysis goes without saying. But there is more. Deleuze and Guattari set us on a path leading to a relationship with the unconscious that is more aligned to the social and political stakes. They strive to articulate an unconscious that does not transcend us in revealing the repressed truth of who we are. Rather, the unconscious that they lay forth is that of an unconscious couched in immanence, thwarting the pitfalls of domination, of expropriation, and of overreach. The goal is to propel the analyst right up to the definitive conclusion of the exercise: "participating in an undertaking that will bring about genuine liberation" rather than running the risk of taking part in "the work of bourgeois repression at its most far-reaching level, that is to say, keeping European humanity harnessed to the yolk of daddy-mommy and *making no effort to do away with this problem once and for all.*"[20]

In this sense, a clinic in a major key would be Freudian, Lacanian, or Kleinian. Or would, in any case, conform to these traditions. It would be undertaken in institutions, on the couch, in therapeutic groups, and in psychoanalytic workshops. What we are referring to is akin to a fortress, replete with crises, with confrontations, with schools, publications, generals and prelates, as well as broadcast media, and failures. Reverberating with reassurance, triumphant, this structure would lay out its laws and hold forth as an arbiter of culture. It would have diagnostic categories at its disposal that are universally applicable for understanding what is at work within each and every subject. The opacity of this structure, and its therapeutic effects, would preclude any substantive questions regarding the political outcomes of its practise. An out-and-out *modus operandi*, a manner of situating both the psychoanalytic position and role.

On the contrary, a clinic in a minor key would be comparable to ways of life which are able to "reopen affective and relational virtualities,"[21] to which Michel Foucault aspired at the end of a striking interview in the French magazine *Gai pied Hebdo*, in 1981 – the year of Lacan's death and at a time when AIDS was not yet known as such, but had already begun to cast its shadow. The clinic in a minor key is another version of the psychoanalytic exercise. It more deeply interrogates the promises made by the psychoanalytic framework and its political consequences. It dares to call into question the legitimacy of certain dogmas: Oedipus, the phallus, the laws of the Symbolic and of castration, as well as the Real as impossible. The clinic in a minor key pushes these dogmas to their very limit so as to understand to what degree, when applied and recited word for word, they result in normative effects, producing the very results that they claim to describe. In other words, a clinic in a minor key does not overlook the fact that the "idea of a program of proposals is dangerous. As soon as a program is presented, it becomes a law, and there's a prohibition against inventing. [...] The program must be wide open."[22]

The clinic in a minor key endeavours, as its name suggests, to undermine the certitudes of the clinic in a major key, scattering these certainties from their well-worn paths. The clinic in a minor key plots their intellectual genealogy. It envisages the body, not as a blank page, upon which the law of the Symbolic is to be applied, but as a locus of tensions, of entanglements that are formed through norms, and as a space where desire erupts, not only in terms of truth as a drive but also in terms of what can today be seen as an extraordinary historical plasticity:

> We have to dig deeply to show how things have been historically contingent, for such and such reason intelligible but not necessary. We must make the intelligible appear against a background of emptiness and deny its necessity. We must think that what exists is far from filling all possible spaces. To make a truly unavoidable challenge of the question: What can be played?[23]

The expression "clinic in a minor key" is the fruit of a strange union. It blends Freudian practice with a concept from Deleuze and Guattari. In their use of the term "minor" Deleuze and Guattari reach out to all those who find themselves powerless and oppressed, to the subalterns, to the downtrodden. The analytical apparatus, such as it has been constructed since Vienna and over the last century, seems, on the contrary, to often address itself to a "major" population: white, heterosexual, dominant.

Again, in other words, a clinic in a minor key designates a field of psychological work pertaining to the unconscious which is open to the demands of minorities. Not to force normality upon these individuals, but to hear them out, understand their differences, and to rethink the apparatus itself using these differences as a starting point. Thus, a clinic in a minor key binds queer critiques of psychoanalysis to its endeavour, not so much as to imagine a psychoanalysis that conforms to minority identity or communitarianism, but rather to interrogate the heteronormative preconceptions of a practice exclusively centred on the question of the phallic and the Oedipal.

Unless one should quite simply say that psychoanalysis has left Vienna behind. That psychoanalysis has set out to read science fiction and had met up with cyborgs?[24] Insist that, no, the hypothesis of the unconscious must not perish. And yet, as a consequence of reciting the Oedipal lesson, of holding too firmly onto the idea of the phallus and the fatherly unconscious, this is no doubt what will happen.

Some history

So as to better understand the ambiguous relation that ties the archipelago of gender theory and more particularly of queer theory to Freud's discoveries let us remember that they have been shaped over a relatively long period of time. The waters in which they bathe have their source in the wake of the medical study of children born "intersex" – these wayward, indecisive and hermaphroditic bodies – to whom John Money – a clinician but not an analyst – applied the social construction of gender identity.[25] The stakes, at the time (during the 1950s), were to consolidate the binary opposition of the sexes from a social and surgical viewpoint. This reflected a vision close to that of Simone de Beauvoir and her famous adage, being a man or being a woman has nothing to do with nature, one becomes oneself culturally as either man or woman. The dualism of the sexes is thus replaced by that of gender.

For their part, gay and lesbian studies appeared as the logical consequence of the communitarian demands and grievances for which the Stonewall riots, on a June 1969 evening in New York remain the most enduring emblem of the fight against the persecution of homosexuals. Such a field of study is, of course, indissociable from the triumphant reception of French Theory in America. On university campuses, homegrown versions and translations of Foucault, Deleuze, Lacan, Derrida and company, appeared: blithely studied, commented and recombined, diffracting both bodies and sexualities.

And then the unwelcome guest showed up. The AIDS crisis threw into sharp relief the degree to which, despite the exuberant experimentation that followed the sexual revolution, and the freedoms that seem to have been acquired, nothing had really moved forward. The dead were left unmourned. The "gay cancer" killed those who, in the opinion of a certain majority, had sought it out. With intelligence, irreverence and in despair, Leo Bersani asked: "Is the rectum a grave?"[26] In such dark times, the criminal indifference when faced with an illness capable of decimating an entire fringe of the population illustrated the blatant heteronormativity of society at large, as well as its underlying, festering, homophobia.

In this context, political, sanitary, medical, and social deadlock had lethal consequences. Refusing to take sides, keeping quiet, or remaining silent (even in terms of the most considerate attention) could not be heard in any way other than that of an astonishing compromise with what some do not hesitate to call a "gay genocide." For the communities involved, the century ended in immense sadness. An anti-homophobic analysis of the manner in which bodies and sexualities had, for the longest time, been conceived, classified and stigmatized was sorely and urgently needed.

An analysis of this kind would result in novel struggles with ethical, political, and even ontological consequences. *The Epistemology of the Closet* by Eve Kosofsky Sedgwick, published in 1990[27] – the same year as the celebrated *Gender Trouble* [28] by Judith Butler – took up this challenge. These publications, together with that of Teresa de Laurentis on the *Technologies of Gender* [29] published three years earlier, gave birth to the queer movement. Queer thought began to assert itself at odds with any identification, be it masculine, feminine, heterosexual, gay, lesbian, bi, or trans. This deregistration from the identificatory index nurtured the proliferation of sexual identities comparable to simulacra without any real consistency: marginal materializations, gender archetypes are no longer binary but are constantly, infinitely, multiplied. As if on stage, they deliver a coterie of colourful characters: femme, butch, transgender, drag-king, drag-queen. So many joyous expressions of the masquerade that underlies the battle of the sexes (here, the plural form is particularly important).

The shores of grievance

In this constellation, psychoanalysis sees itself, at times, accused of heteronormativity, while at others, accused of being a "feminist theory *manqué*"[30] either supposed to rectify the "disorder and illogic of desires with health, purity and stability,"[31] or belittled as being subject to the (bio-) power of the body, to practices and to desire, or even simply ridiculed.[32] Certain statements, separated from their context are dissected and sparkle with latent or explicit homophobia. It is nevertheless striking to note how these theories feed on the contributions of analytic knowledge: the plasticity of the drives, the influence that language has on our bodies, the openness to and the dependence upon Alterity are all among the themes that crisscross the work of queer theorists, postfeminists, and the more recent field of porn studies.[33]

The proto-queer theorist Monique Wittig laid the foundations for these critiques of psychoanalysis. In the course of a career straddling both France and the United States, her academic work goes against the structuralism of Claude Lévi-Strauss and Lacanian psychoanalysis. Her key essay, "The Straight Mind" responds, beginning with its title, to the essay "The Savage Mind" by Lévi-Strauss. For Wittig, the psychoanalyst extorts a truth capable of pathologizing the homosexual subject – the praxis deprives the subject of his speech. Both the subject's speech and his actions are thus no longer seen as anything other than symptoms. She drives home her proposition in stating:

> People who did not fall into the power of the psychoanalytical institution may experience an immeasurable feeling of sadness at the degree of oppression (of manipulation) that the psychoanalyzed discourses show. In the analytical experience there is an oppressed person, the psychoanalyzed, whose need for communication is exploited and who (in the same way as the witches could, under torture, only repeat the language that the inquisitors wanted to hear) has no other choice, (if s/he does not

> want to destroy the implicit contract which allows her/him to communicate and which s/he needs), than to attempt to say what s/he is supposed to say. They say that this can last for a lifetime [...][34]

Braced by the interpretation of the unconscious, the analyst contributes to hiding from the view of the oppressed the "material cause of their oppression and plunges them into a kind of ahistoric vacuum."[35] Under these conditions, advances in gender and queer theories in the wake of Wittig, would correspond to the possibility of reappropriating an understanding, notably of homosexuality, that psychoanalysis would have, in part, monopolized, in explaining and in expropriating a space in which the self can both be considered and formulated. More recently, taking the evolutions and the advances of the homosexual movements into account, the sociologist Eric Fassin pinpointed, in his expression "inversion of the homosexual question," the refusal to be dispossessed of self-formulation. As he states, "generally, it is not so much society that questions homosexuality, than homosexuality that subjects society to an interrogation."[36] With the emergence of communitarian thought, psychoanalysis would have lost its capacity to analyse homosexualities: "Who are you?"; "Why are you here?"; "What do you represent?"; "How do you come about?"... These questions have progressively lost all meaning. Those most involved prefer, as the case may be, to ask these questions with their own words and to answer them in the same manner. Little by little, this reversal would come about, not only in the field of homosexualities but also for each sexual specificity, for each imaginary identification, in short, for all forms of gender identity. However, if this identitarian understanding has taken root in LGBTQI+[37] communities as well as in the related academic, militant, and ideological domains, it is clear that such freedoms of self-definition turn out to be far from settled in a broader social sense.

Thus laid out, the mobile archipelago of gender and queer theory with its unstable contours and sometimes violent undercurrents can have a substantial effect on the analyst's discourse: better pin down the place that the analyst occupies, reformulate the ins and outs of its singular ethics. It is no longer a question of speaking "for," or of defining what such and such sexual minorities are. Each of them are quite capable of finding the words to express what they feel, experience, or think that they are. On the contrary, and much more simply, in the litany of grievances that have been broadly addressed to psychoanalysis, new considerations of style and substance have seen the light of day: to hear and understand the wounds and oppressions, to offer a space in which these wounds can be (re)dressed, to accommodate vulnerability and to work to transform it into strength. These modest and certainly respectful perspectives, open-endedly outline the scope of a new clinic in a minor key.

A double opportunity?

When Lacan carried out his "return to Freud,"[38] he continually and rigorously illustrated the logic at work in the unconscious. The de-constructions arising out of queer theory, gay and lesbian studies, and out of gender theory took up the genealogies established by Foucault, questioning the unconscious, undermining this very logic. These movements sought, and quite rightly so, to situate this logic in its time frame. Are the forms and conceptual tools that, today still, guide the cure – developmental stages, phallus, Woman, jouissance, castration, complex or drive, etc. – not themselves inscribed in the history of thought or do they possess an otherwise eternal effectiveness? Can the semantic shifts from the biological to the symbolic be subject to critique? Does the exemplification of "sexual maturity," of development which typically results in the "genital stage,"[39] of the choice of the heterosexual subject and the (re-)production of a family-centric model able to offer the subject something to "love and work on,"[40] still manage to grasp what is embodied, said, and experienced by contemporary subjects?

At a time when strict representations, binary opposition and biological certitudes falter, is an update of the psychoanalytic lexicon not precisely what is called for? Unless, at the very least, it suffices to cite clinical work, the specificity of the cure, so as to deflect from political mirages and return to the private experience of psychological life? Faced with these questions, sometimes asked in urgency, sometimes violently, how can psychoanalysis justify itself? Should psychoanalysis respond to the supposed deficiencies that have been ascribed to it? Or, on the contrary, can the century-old and affably attentive discipline allow itself to remain, always and forever, cloistered in an interpretative silence? For Eric Fassin:

> it is always for psychoanalysis to determine, not only if it should move, but how it should move – that is to say, that it is up to psychoanalysts, if they deem it to be a good time, to determine the new paths that their discipline will take [...] For the most part, the work remains to be done.[41]

Later, Fassin leaves the path open for a reinvention of the praxis, on the condition that women's liberation, together with that of all the minor peoples be understood as having already taken place from both a theoretical and a behavioural point of view. In other words, the feminist and post-feminist deconstructions have succeeded, together with the parallel development of the pharmaceutical toolkit and modern medical imaging, in endangering psychoanalytic theory.

Paradoxically, this perhaps represents a double opportunity for psychoanalysis. On the one hand, the work of theoretic deconstruction undertaken by the field of cultural studies represents an opportunity for psychoanalysis to disentangle the complexities of its own tools. On the other hand, that analytical practice is to be confronted by its own therapeutic failure, is not new. It would be illusory to think that an analysis that has been concluded is synonymous with a cure. In *Further Recommendations on the Technique of Psycho-Analysis* Freud warned against the *furor sanadi.* [42] Psychoanalysis does not aim at curing everything in a flash. Recall that in *Analysis Terminable and Interminable*, psychoanalysis is qualified as an impossible profession in which the analyst is constantly confronted by their own failure.[43] The patient's resistance when faced with the cure is infinite. This degree of modesty as concerns the success of the undertaking constitutes a recurring theme in Freud's work. This should not only be seen in terms of a form of renunciation of an eventual betterment of the patient. Failure propels the practice itself. Freud's interest in the death drive as an essential force of the human psyche prevents him from falling into a well-meaning teleological illusion of finality, of a successful cure as defined by a perfect readaptation to social norms. It is thus clear that the analysis, contrary to any life coaching, or the practise of positive thinking, is radically propelled by frustration, failure, and fundamental incompletion.

This is a substantial paradox, but one which it is better to own up to: contrary to derivative psychologizing that unrelentingly aims at rectifying behaviour, psychoanalysis does not target the patient's well-being but rather his desire and his jouissance. The stakes are infinitely more far reaching and complex than behaviour which is adequately conformist, an obsessive-compulsive disorder that is mastered, or anxiety that is managed. The strength of desire is to be intimately tied to that part of our psyche which is darkest, most destructive, least approving, and least logical: *jouissance.* "What is jouissance? Here it amounts to no more than a negative instance. Jouissance is what serves no purpose."[44]

Without a doubt, rereading certain of Freud's statements, together with his belief in biology as the foundation of his interpretation, offers a nearly inexhaustible font from which critiques can be drawn by those theoreticians who seek to deconstruct gender. This major figure in psychoanalysis is not without his difficulties. But beyond this conservative caricature, blatantly affirming that "for the psychical field, the biological field does in fact play the part of the underlying bedrock,"[45] lies the Freud of the death drive. Freud, in his writings, skirted the very edge of this unsettling phenomenon, which Lacan later gave a central role through his use of the notion of jouissance. From this, the impossibility of analysis as a profession can be deduced: "the death instinct, [...] the urge of what is living to return to an inanimate state"[46] is a strange companion. Insatiable troublemaker. Unique discovery. Intolerably shattering meaning and sense.

Psychoanalysis has never worked as such. It does not want to heal the subjects it encounters. There is no "therapeutic" analysis even if the psychoanalytic process well and truly inspires genuine therapeutic effects. Moreover, the aforementioned deconstructions could certainly benefit somewhat from focusing less on the aspect of logical sense than on the outside-of-sense that psychoanalysis foregrounds. What we encounter in the psychoanalytic practice, what we are confronted with, is, in effect, an outside-of-sense, an adaptation of sorts to proper functioning, to the correct sequencing or organization of the world, something beyond the pleasure principle.[47] In the course of analysis we don't build on any techniques or tricks to encourage well-being. We cast ourselves off. We lose ourselves. We undo ourselves. We seize onto that which is singular, which pulls us towards a future, an alteration of the self, a release from the rational, educable, adaptive, assessable Ego.

All types of (gender) inversions!

In a pamphlet railing against psychoanalysis, philosopher and historian Didier Éribon, celebrated trend setter in gay studies and queer theory, was saddened by the mysterious way in which certain of the most eminent exponents of "radical thought – feminist, gay and lesbian, queer – continue to refer to psychoanalytic theories as if it was possible to reformulate these theories in a non-normative sense."[48] While at first blush, certain of the deconstructions undertaken by partisans of gender studies virulently lay into the analytic praxis, Éribon highlights the inverse: queer theory has closely read psychoanalysis, and would have been better served by ignoring it!

Éribon explains that a critical discourse, unmasking the social and cognitive structures which fetter individual freedom, would allow individuals to be happy. Those who have experienced a psychoanalytic cure cannot but attest to the optimism of this line of reasoning. When we accept the paradox of healing as absent, we refuse any psychological "orthopaedics"[49] of speech and of Ego. The subject who gives themselves unto the analytic couch never finds a discourse which perfectly suits him. He learns to live with the fundamental inadequacy that marks the distance between his body and language. He is equally unable to name his desire as he is to prevent himself from being unsettled by his jouissance. Such is the motor of the analytic procedure: no sublimation without failure, no sense without a flight from sense, no affirmation without negation, no desire without jouissance.

Meanwhile Éribon asks himself "if it is truly possible – and desirable – to set oneself a project that aims to bring together queer theory, or in a more general manner, radical thought, by one name or another, [...] and psychoanalysis."[50] The philosopher had great difficulties with the fact that Judith Butler, who is no doubt one of the most well-known gender theorists, considers "through Freud, that which could be lacking in Foucault's theory of power, that is to say a theory of the manner in which power functions in the individual psyche."[51] This is however the most interesting aspect of Butler's work, as well as of those who, in her wake, "reformulate the key notions of the analytic doctrine, thus rendering them compatible with the multiple realities of desire, fantasy, identity, and affective, sexual and familial arrangements, in short, the lives that individuals in their inalienable diversity live."[52]

Gayle Rubin, anthropologist, postfeminist, critical and attentive reader of Lacan and another cornerstone of queer theory, considers the goal of her research to be the creation of a "society without gender,"[53] that is to say a "feminist revolution [that] would liberate more than women. It would liberate forms of sexual expression, and it would liberate human personality from the straitjacket of gender."[54] In order to achieve her project, the author does not hesitate to affirm the absolute necessity of taking psychoanalysis into account: "dismissing it would be suicidal for a political movement dedicated to eradicating gender hierarchy (or gender itself). We cannot dismantle something that we underestimate or do not understand."[55]

Minor people's interest in psychoanalysis is not secondary: it is a question of survival. In the analytic field as in that of gender deconstruction, language is tied to the body through sexuality. The clinical approach connects sexuality to the drives and to the libidinal flows. Queer studies, in turn, attaches sexuality to the social and to the political. In either case, sex is no longer biological, it is removed from the reproductive sphere so as to ally the intimate either to language or to politics.

As a consequence of seeking too keenly to "escape psychoanalysis," Éribon concludes by calling into question the radical thought that is the subject of his consideration, preferring to cloister himself in the history of philosophy as a field of study, at the risk of overlooking the former's micropolitical scope. In his opinion it is better to reconcile Sartre and Foucault than to read Freud or Lacan! At this juncture we understand that: instead of putting up with the real, the anxiety and the suffering at work both in the preoccupations of minorities as well as in the quotidian of the clinic, Éribon elects to steadfastly remain in the realm of the history of ideas. And yet, in the ideological domain as well as in that of sexual activism, this realm of abstraction and ethereal reflection is left behind in lieu of alternate engagements. In the same way, but by other means, in psychoanalysis we also tie ourselves to that which is concrete: we choose to pinpoint, on a case-by-case basis, that which rings hollow in a given subject without regard for their sexual proclivities. Either way, the real takes precedence over the ideal.

The clinic in a minor key does not opt for a revolutionary utopianism. Following Lacan's lead, it is concerned with the modes of jouissance in which the subject immerses itself. In lieu of proposing a systematic deconstruction of identity (or identities) while waiting for a future paradise, or alternately, mourning the loss of the symbolic order while hoping for the triumphant return of the Name-of-the-Father, the psychoanalytic clinic identifies that which, endlessly, repeats itself and precludes an encounter with Desire, which for each and every one of us, in an irremediably different manner, strains the fullness of meaning. The psychoanalytic clinic is, in essence, a space for questioning, where we can rework, tinker with, and reassemble in words that which refuses to enter into definitive and secure categories.

But if psychoanalysis is already so subversive, why should it engage with the work of queer studies? Not only because the latter refers to psychoanalysis, but also in so far as it addresses psychoanalysis. It informs psychoanalysis that it has overlooked the consequences of the discovery of libidinal life. In her 1975 essay "The Traffic in Women," Gayle Rubin offers this lapidary judgement: "Psychoanalysis is a feminist theory *manquée*."[56] For her, the rejection of Freud by the women's and gay movements has its roots "in the rejection by psychoanalysis of its own insights."[57] It is difficult not to consider this critique in light of that rendered by Deleuze and Guattari several years prior in *Anti-Oedipus*. They explain that "Freud made the most profound discovery of the abstract subjective essence of desire –Libido. But since he realienated this essence, reinvesting it in a subjective system of representation of the ego."[58] In so far as Gayle Rubin considers that psychoanalysis has not sufficiently taken women's struggles, from a political-social point of view, into account, Deleuze and Guattari begrudge the cowardliness of psychoanalysis. Psychoanalysis recoils when faced with the social and political consequences of its ethical position.

The discovery of the unconscious and of the libido were a first step towards the abolition of gender in society. This is why those who seek to conclude this struggle should not ignore psychoanalysis. Besides, given a paradox capable of undermining common sense, aimed both at the subject's desire and their death drive, sounding the unconscious, hearing that which "doesn't stop not being written,"[59] would logically have defied reproductive conservatism, well-meaning moralism, and beliefs which exclusively promote the heterosexual family.

As clinicians, in order to be able to address the real as it erupts into contemporary life, we have to take these critiques into account. But answering queer and minor communities does not merely consist of searching for elements that would remedy the postfeminist "shortcomings" of psychoanalysis. Nor would it consist of returning to a pre- or anti-Oedipal reality. The analytic response brings about another kind of responsibility. Better to explain how the praxis, the encounter with the unconscious dimension, the undertaking of the drive, takes the real into account in so far as it manifests differently for each subject, that is to say by disrupting the intelligibility of social grievances, however well justified.

If the queer community were to speak to psychoanalysis, how could they be answered? What can be done in order to work through desire without silencing the postfeminists and their just demands? It is true that the clinical practice puts militantism on hold, but this is not so much a result of a "lack of vision" as it is out of concern for the real and the distress which dwells within the subject. If the struggle for the recognition of equal rights is necessary for the construction of morally emancipated subjectivities, it does not suffice for the liberation of these self-same subjects caught up in failings of the sexual order. Herein lies psychoanalytic responsibility. Whatever our proclivities or practices, heterosexual, homosexual, or even naught,[60] and whatever the degree of permissibility present within the society within which we find ourselves, even in the most harmonious and egalitarian of utopias, as a subject of the unconscious we will always be afflicted, in our own way, by the short-circuit between words and jouissance.

In opposition to other therapeutic practices within the field of mental health, psychoanalysis does not rehabilitate the subject in order to ensure optimal functioning. Psychoanalysis does not seek to optimize the efficiency of its care. It gives expression to a dimension other than those which prevail in society at large. Without a doubt, analysis remains one of the rare spaces – perhaps the only space – where the subject is empowered to take hold of the difficulty of (his or her) being in a singularly authentic manner, without necessary recourse to any authorization other than that which the subject offers him- or herself. The analytic trajectory may seem surprising: it disrupts the universal, refuses the construction of individualisms, suspends conformity, liberating the subject in unexpected ways. Cold comfort for those who await a better world, this humble first step leads less to a pluralistic struggle than to an irreducible self.

Dislodging the four poles

It is quite clear that two versions of psychoanalysis face each other in opposition. One hermeneutic and one therapeutic, one attached to the symbolic and the other to the real, one to politics and the other to the intimate, to language and to the body, to the signifier and the drives. This vision further opposes a consideration of psychoanalysis as an unavoidable point of reference for feminism to that of its inescapable sworn enemy, as conservative bulwark in terms of social norms and its ardent critic, the major key and the minor key. In examining this network of tensions, in consolidating and in unwinding them, we will, no doubt, learn more about the specificity of psychoanalysis itself and about certain silences that endure within the discipline.

At bottom, queer communities writ large can be seen to articulate four fundamental grievances as concerns psychoanalysis. These interlocking critiques spiral inexorably from one to the other coalescing into a sort of a four-poled structure as unwieldy as it is violent, as deaf as it is imposing. I am not seeking to show that these antipsychoanalytic grievances miss their target. On the contrary, I believe that their aim is true. Psychoanalysis, in taking these critiques into account, in hearing them out, in modulating its attention, in appreciating their implications as concerns both practice and metapsychology could, at once, continue to assume the specificity that is particular to psychoanalysis, and explicitly demonstrate its openness to "becoming-minor."[61] With these four grievances, given a commitment to dislodging their structure, I will neither deplore the collapse of the symbolic order, nor rejoice at scientific capitalist omnipotence or so-called progress (technological, biological, pharmaceutical…). Rather, it is a question of confronting the real in so far as it asserts itself and to which minorities of all shapes and forms can testify.

Let us map out these four poles of grievance. The analytic dispositive, governed by the "profound and universal power"[62] of the Oedipal law (chapter II) which underscores at once the homophobia (chapter III) and the heteronormativity (chapter IV) at work in society more broadly, and which precludes moving beyond sexual difference (chapter V). Oedipal, homophobic, heteronormative, and attached to a binary representation of the sexes, thus conceived, psychoanalysis would fail subjects whose identities, practices, acts, modes of relating, forms of love, and even whose bodies do not conform to the expectations of the Viennese turn-of-the-century petty bourgeoisie.

These four grievances rhythm the chapters that follow. For each of the critiques it is necessary to reconcile the ins and outs of the dispositive. Dislodging the four poles of grievance is not a thankless task, it affords us the opportunity to consider, that, in light of the theories of gender deconstruction, things do not, or no longer, work, they do not operate as they should. This is the equivalent of having a thorn in one's side: the analytic apparatus does not function as it should, it prevents us from calmly continuing our clinical activity, it represents a wakeup call.

Four questions thus direct our undertaking here. How to move beyond the Oedipal structure? Does homo-analysis exist? Can the psychic structure be elaborated in terms other than those of heterosexual norms? Should our approach to the unconscious be mediated by the biological and social "fact" that there are two, and only two, sexes?

Notes

1 In reference to Michel Foucault's analysis of the literary and critical works of Maurice Blanchot. See Michel Foucault, "Maurice Blanchot: The Thought from Outside," *Foucoult Blanchot*, trans. Brian Massumi (Zone Books, 1987).

2 For an excellent reconsideration of this concept see Sabine Prokhoris, *L'Insaisissable Histoire de la Psychanalyse*, Presses Universitaires de France, 2014.

3 Speaking of gender studies as a singular notion gives the impression that it represents a unified field of thought whereas one should, in essence, consider the plurality of the various theories at work, as Judith Butler reminds us. See Judith Butler, "Genre et théorie: Judith Butler nous écrit," *Le Nouvel Obs*, February 10, 2014, https://www.nouvelobs.com/essais/20140210.OBS5705/genre-et-theorie-judith-butler-nous-ecrit.html.

4 This is a reference to Édouard Molinaro's 1978 film, *La Cage Aux Folles* [The Birdcage]. In his comprehensive study of the history of cinema and homosexuality, Didier Roth-Bettoni offers a fresh analysis of the clichés that, for the longest time, have been the stock and trade of popular cinema. See Didier Roth-Bettoni, *L'Homosexualité au cinema*, Paris, La Musardine, 2007, pp. 243–244.

5 This is what Beatriz Paul Preciado illustrates in "Sex design," an essay which was published in *Airs de Paris* (the catalogue of the exhibition that was presented by the Centre Pompidou, in Gallery 1 from 25 April to 16 August 2007). See Beatriz Paul Preciado, "Sex design," in *Airs de Paris*, ed. Valérie Guillaume and Christine Marcel (Éditions du Centre Pompidou, 2007).
6 The way in which the body, and the female body in particular, has been constructed and "pathologized," notably by the dildo, is constitutive of an especially important field of study. See Rachel P. Maines, *The Technology of Orgasm: "Hysteria," the Vibrator, and Women's Sexual Satisfaction*, (Johns Hopkins University Press, 1999) and Georges Didi-Huberman, *Invention of Hysteria*, trans. Alisa Hartz (MIT Press, 2003).
7 Beatriz Preciado, *Testo Junkie: Sex, Drugs and Biopolitics in the Pharmacopornographic Era*, trans. Bruce Benderson (The Feminist Press, 2013), 379–380.
8 Thamy Ayouch has also used this distinction in a number of academic articles wherein he refers to a "major psychoanalysis" and a "minor psychoanalysis." While I feel an intellectual kinship and proximity to his line of thought, I nevertheless feel that this question is better considered through the lens of the clinic, in the specificity that is proper to the encounter between two subjects, in that which is constructed, not merely in terms of metapsychological concepts and their theoretical deconstruction, but in intimate proximity to a lived experience shared with minor peoples. See Thamy Ayouch, "Genre, classe, race et subalternité: pour une psychanalyse mineur," in *Pour un regard neuf de la psychanalyse sur le genre et la parentalité*, ed. Laurence Croix and Gérard Pommier (Editions Eres, 2018), 185. See also Thamy Ayouch, "Sexe et genre sur le divan ou pour une psychanalyse mineur" foreword to *Sexe et genre sur le divan. Théories du sexuel dans le discours de la clinique psy en France contemporaine* by Thiphaine Besnard-Santini (L'Harmattan, 2017) as well as Thamy Ayouch, *Psychanalyse et hybridité. Genre, colonialité, subjectivation* (Leuven University Press, 2018).
9 Gilles Deleuze and Félix Guattari, *Kafka: Toward a Minor Literature*, trans. Dana Polan (University of Minnesota Press, 1986), 19.
10 Gilles Deleuze and Félix Guattari, *A Thousand Plateaus. Capitalism and Schizophrenia*, trans. Brian Massumi (University of Minnesota Press, 1987), 76.
11 Deleuze and Guattari, *A Thousand Plateaus*, 101.
12 Deleuze and Guattari, *Kafka: Toward a Minor Literature*, 23.
13 Deleuze and Guattari, *A Thousand Plateaus*, 97.
14 Deleuze and Guattari, *A Thousand Plateaus*, 97.
15 Deleuze and Guattari, *A Thousand Plateaus*, 106.
16 Which I develop in the following chapter.
17 Jacques Lacan, "Variations on the Standard Treatment" in *Écrits*, trans. Bruce Fink (W.W. Norton & Company, 2006), 298.
18 Jacques Lacan, "Variations on the Standard Treatment," 290.
19 Jacques Lacan, "Variations on the Standard Treatment," 297.
20 Gilles Deleuze and Félix Guattari, *Anti-Oedipus. Capitalism and Schizophrenia*, trans. Robert Hurley, Mark Seem and Helen R. Lane (University of Minnesota Press, 1983), 50.
21 Michel Foucault, "Friendship as a Way of Life" in *Ethics, Subjectivity and Truth: The Essential Works of Michel Foucault 1954–1984, Volume I*, ed. Paul Rabinow, trans. Robert Hurley and John Johnston (The New Press, 1997), 138.
22 Michel Foucault, "Friendship as a Way of Life," 139.
23 Michel Foucault, "Friendship as a Way of Life," 139–140.
24 For a feminist consideration of cyborgs and a reflection on the new forms of resistance and subjectivity through technology, see Donna Haraway "A Cyborg

Manifesto: Science, Technology, and Socialist-Feminism in the Late Twentieth Century" in *Simians, Cyborgs, and Women: The Reinvention of Nature* (Routledge, 1991). See also the excellent introduction to this line of political technologist thought in Thierry Hoquet, *Cyborg philosophie. Penser contre les dualisms* (Seuil, 2011).

25 For an introduction to theories of gender and their history as well as for a perspective on the notion of gender as a conceptual tool at work within numerous disciplines see Laurie Laufer and Florence Rochefort, *Qu'est-ce que le genre?* (Payot, 2014).

26 Leo Bersani, "Is the Rectum a Grave?" in *Is the Rectum a Grave? And Other Essays* (University of Chicago Press, 2010), 3 – 30.

27 Eve Kosofsky Sedgwick, *Epistemology of the Closet* (University of California Press, 1990).

28 Judith Butler, *Gender Trouble: Feminism and the Subversion of Identity* (Routledge, 1990).

29 Teresa de Laurentis, "The Technology of Gender" in *Technologies of Gender: Essays on Theory, Film and Fiction* (Indiana University Press, 1987), 1–31.

30 Gayle Rubin "The Traffic in Women: Notes on the Political Economy of Sex" in *Toward an Anthropology of Women*, ed. Rayna R. Reiter, (Monthly Review Press, 1975), 185.

31 Judith Halberstam and Ira Livingston, "Introduction: Posthuman Bodies" in *Posthuman Bodies*, ed. Judith Halberstam and Ira Livingston (Indiana University Press, 1995), 13.

32 In France, Marie-Hélène Sam Bourcier, who is today known as Sam Bourcier, and who identifies as male, has raised this subject to an art form. See Marie-Hélène Sam Bourcier, *Queer Zone. Politique des identités sexuelles, des representations et des savoirs* (Editions Amsterdam, 2006) as well as Marie-Hélène Sam Bourcier, *Queer Zone 2* (Editions Amsterdam, 2006) and Marie-Hélène Sam Bourcier, *Queer Zone 3* (Editions Amsterdam, 2006). See also, Sam Bourcier, *Homo Inc.orporated. Le triangle et La licorne qui pète* (Calbourakis, 2017). See also an excerpt which has been translated into English via the Italian translation: Sandra D'Urso, "On Translation: 'Homo Inc.orporated: The Triangle and the Farting Unicorn'" in *The Palgrave Handbook of Queer and TransFeminisms in Contemporary Performance*, ed. Tiina Rosenberg, Sandra D'Urso, Anna Renée Winget, (Palgrave Macmillan, 2021), 63–78.

33 Regarding this field of study, see the excellent anthology: Florian Voros (ed.), *Cultures pornographiques. Anthologie des Porn studies* (Editions Amsterdam, 2015).

34 Monique Wittig, "The Straight Mind" in *The Straight Mind and Other Essays* (Beacon Press, 1992), 23.

35 Monique Wittig, "The Straight Mind," 22.

36 "De manière générale, ce n'est plus tant la société qui interroge l'homosexualité, que l'homosexualité qui soumet la societé à la question." Eric Fassin, *L'Inversion de la question homosexuelle* (Editions Amsterdam, 2008), 17.

37 This acronym signifies Lesbian, Gay, Bi, Trans, Queer, and Intersex persons, with the + signifying an openness to the multitudes that wish to express their gender in an alternate fashion.

38 See Jacques Lacan, "The Function and Field of Speech and Language in Psychoanalysis" in *Écrits*, trans. Bruce Fink (W.W. Norton & Company, 2006), 221.

39 These are recurrent terms in Freud and the post-Freudians. As concerns homosexuality see, for example, Sigmund Freud, "Five Lectures on Psycho-analysis" in *The Standard Edition of the Complete Psychological Works of Sigmund Freud*. Vol. XI. Edited by James Strachey, Anna Freud, and Angela Richards. (Hogarth Press, 1953 - 1974), 44–46.

40 See Sigmund Freud, "Civilization and its Discontents" in *The Standard Edition of the Complete Psychological Works of Sigmund Freud.* Vol. XXI, 101.
41 "c'est toutefois à la psychanalyse de determiner non seulement *si* elle doit bouger, mais *comment* elle doit bouger – c'est-à-dire qu'il appartient aux psychanalystes, s'ils le jugent bon, de determiner les voies nouvelles qu'empruntera leur discipline. [...] Pour l'essentiel, le travail reste à faire." Eric Fassin, *L'Inversion de la question homosexuelle,* 210.
42 Sigmund Freud, "Observations on Transference-Love (Further Recomendations on the Technique of Psycho-Analysis III)" in *The Standard Edition of the Complete Psychological Works of Sigmund Freud.* Vol. XII, 171. See also the work of Paul-Laurent Assoun regarding this important warning that Freud gives us, see Paul-Laurent Assoun, "Du métier impossible à l'acte necessaire. L'effet analytique" *Figures de la psychanalyse* 1, no. 15 (2007): 17–31, doi: 10.3917/fp.015.0017.
43 Sigmund Freud, "Analysis Terminable and Interminable" in *The Standard Edition of the Complete Psychological Works of Sigmund Freud.* Vol. XXIII, 248.
44 Jacques Lacan, *The Seminar of Jacques Lacan. On Feminine Sexuality, The Limits of Love and Knowledge,* Book XX, ed. Jacques-Alain Miller, trans. Bruce Fink (W. W. Norton & Company, 1998), 3.
45 Sigmund Freud, "Analysis Terminable and Interminable" in *The Standard Edition of the Complete Psychological Works of Sigmund Freud.* Vol. XXIII, 252.
46 Sigmund Freud, "Analysis Terminable and Interminable" in *The Standard Edition of the Complete Psychological Works of Sigmund Freud.* Vol. XXIII, 246.
47 Sigmund Freud, "Beyond the Pleasure Principle" in *The Standard Edition of the Complete Psychological Works of Sigmund Freud.* Vol. XVIII, 7–67.
48 "La pensée radicale – feministe, gay et lesbienne, *queer* – continuai[en]t de se référer aux theories psychanalytiques, comme s'il était possible de reformuler celles-ci dans un sens non-normatif." Didier Éribon, *Échapper à la psychanalyse* (Léo Scheer, 2005), 12.
49 Jacques Lacan, "The Function and Field of Speech and Language in Psychoanalysis" in *Écrits,* 251.
50 "s'il est vraiment possible – et souhaitable – de se donner comme projet de rapprocher la théorie *queer,* ou, d'une manière plus générale, la pensée radicale, quell que soit le nom qu'on veuille lui donner, [...] de la psychanalyse." Didier Éribon, *Échapper à la psychanalyse,* 81.
51 "par l'intermédiaire de Freud, ce qui manquerait à la théorie foucaldienne du pouvoir, c'est-à-dire une théorie de la manière dont le pouvoir fonctionne dans le psychisme individuel." Didier Éribon, *Échapper à la psychanalyse,* 82.
52 "reformuler les notions clés de la doctrine analytique afin de les render compatibles avec la réalité multiple des désirs, des fantasmes, des identités, des arrangements affectifs, sexuels, familiaux, bref, des vies que vivent les individus dans leur inalienable diversité." Didier Éribon, *Échapper à la psychanalyse,* 83.
53 Gayle Rubin "The Traffic in Women: Notes on the Political Economy of Sex," 157.
54 Gayle Rubin "The Traffic in Women: Notes on the Political Economy of Sex," 200.
55 Gayle Rubin "The Traffic in Women: Notes on the Political Economy of Sex," 198.
56 Gayle Rubin "The Traffic in Women: Notes on the Political Economy of Sex," 185.
57 Gayle Rubin "The Traffic in Women: Notes on the Political Economy of Sex," 184.
58 Gilles Deleuze and Félix Guattari, *Anti-Oedipus. Capitalism and Schizophrenia,* 333.
59 Jacques Lacan, *The Seminar of Jacques Lacan. On Feminine Sexuality, The Limits of Love and Knowledge,* Book XX, 94.
60 As highlighted by Peggy Sastre, *No Sex. Avoir envie de ne pas faire l'amour* (La Musardine, 2010).

61 This turn of phrase is drawn from the work of Deleuze and Guattari – I will come back to this expression in the following chapter.
62 Sigmund Freud, "The Interpretation of Dreams" in *The Standard Edition of the Complete Psychological Works of Sigmund Freud*. Vol. IV, 261.

Bibliography

Assoun, Paul-Laurent. "Du métier impossible à l'acte necessaire. L'effet analytique." *Figures de la psychanalyse* 1, no. 15 (2007): 17–31. doi: doi:10.3917/fp.015.0017.

Ayouch, Thamy. "Sexe et genre sur le divan ou pour une psychanalyse mineur." Foreword to *Sexe et genre sur le divan. Théories du sexuel dans le discours de la Clinique psy en France contemporaine* by Thiphaine Besnard-Santini. L'Harmattan, 2017.

Ayouch, Thamy. "Genre, classe, race et subalternité: pour une psychanalyse mineur." In *Pour un regard neuf de la psychanalyse sur le genre et la parentalité*. Edited by Laurence Croix and Gérard Pommier, 185–216. Editions Eres, 2018.

Ayouch, Thamy. *Psychanalyse et hybridité. Genre, colonialité, subjectivation*. Leuven University Press, 2018.

Bersani, Leo. "Is the Rectum a Grave?" In *Is the Rectum a Grave? And Other Essays.* University of Chicago Press, 2010.

Bourcier, Marie-Hélène Sam. *Queer Zone. Politique des identités sexuelles, des representations et des savoirs.* Editions Amsterdam, 2006.

Bourcier, Marie-Hélène Sam. *Queer Zone 2*. Editions Amsterdam, 2006.

Bourcier, Marie-Hélène Sam. *Queer Zone 3*. Editions Amsterdam, 2006.

Bourcier, Sam. *Homo Inc.orporated. Le triangle et La licorne qui pète.* Calbourakis, 2017.

Butler, Judith. *Gender Trouble: Feminism and the Subversion of Identity.* Routledge, 1990.

Butler, Judith. "Genre et théorie: Judith Butler nous écrit," *Le Nouvel Obs.* February 10, 2014. https://www.nouvelobs.com/essais/20140210.OBS5705/genre-et-theorie-judith-butler-nous-ecrit.html.

de Laurentis, Teresa. "The Technology of Gender." In *Technologies of Gender: Essays on Theory, Film and Fiction*. Indiana University Press, 1987.

D'Urso, Sandra. "On Translation: 'Homo Inc.orporated: The Triangle and the Farting Unicorn'." In *The Palgrave Handbook of Queer and TransFeminisms in Contemporary Performance.* Edited by Tiina Rosenberg, Sandra D'Urso, and Anna Renée Winget, 63–78. Palgrave Macmillan, 2021.

Deleuze, Gilles and Félix Guattari, *Anti-Oedipus. Capitalism and Schizophrenia.* Translated by Robert Hurley, Mark Seem, and Helen R. Lane. University of Minnesota Press, 1983.

Deleuze, Gilles and Félix Guattari. *Kafka: Toward a Minor Literature.* Translated by Dana Polan. University of Minnesota Press, 1986.

Deleuze, Gilles and Félix Guattari. *A Thousand Plateaus. Capitalism and Schizophrenia.* Translated by Brian Massumi. University of Minnesota Press, 1987.

Didi-Huberman, Georges. *Invention of Hysteria*. Translated by Alisa Hartz. MIT Press, 2003.

Éribon, Didier. *Échapper à la psychanalyse.* Léo Scheer, 2005.

Fassin, Eric. *L'Inversion de la question homosexuelle.* Editions Amsterdam, 2008.

Foucault, Michel. "Maurice Blanchot: The Thought from Outside." In *Foucoult Blanchot*. Translated by Brian Massumi. Zone Books, 1987.

Foucault, Michel. "Friendship as a Way of Life." In *Ethics, Subjectivity and Truth: The Essential Works of Michel Foucault 1954–1984*, Volume I. Edited by Paul Rabinow. Translated by Robert Hurley and John Johnston. The New Press, 1997.

Freud, Sigmund. *The Standard Edition of the Complete Psychological Works of Sigmund Freud.* Edited by James Strachey, Anna Freud, and Angela Richards. Hogarth Press, 1953–1974.

Halberstam, Judith and Ira Livingston. "Introduction: Posthuman Bodies." In *Posthuman Bodies.* Edited by Judith Halberstam and Ira Livingston. Indiana University Press, 1995.

Haraway, Donna J. "A Cyborg Manifesto: Science, Technology, and Socialist-Feminism in the Late Twentieth Century." In *Simians, Cyborgs, and Women: The Reinvention of Nature.* Routledge, 1991.

Hoquet, Thierry. *Cyborg philosophie. Penser contre les dualisms.* Seuil, 2011.

Lacan, Jacques. *On Feminine Sexuality, The Limits of Love and Knowledge. The Seminar of Jacques Lacan.* Book XX. Edited by Jacques-Alain Miller. Translated by Bruce Fink. W.W. Norton & Company, 1998.

Lacan, Jacques. *Écrits.* Translated by Bruce Fink. W.W. Norton & Company, 2006.

Laufer, Laurie and Florence Rochefort. *Qu'est-ce que le genre?*Payot, 2014.

Maines, Rachel P. *The Technology of Orgasm: "Hysteria," the Vibrator, and Women's Sexual Satisfaction.* John Hopkins University Press, 1999.

Molinaro, Édouard. *La Cage Aux Folles.* United Artists, 1978.

Preciado, Beatriz Paul. "Sex design." In *Airs de Paris*, edited by Valérie Guillaume and Christine Marcel. Éditions du Centre Pompidou, 2007.

Preciado, Beatriz. *Testo Junkie: Sex, Drugs and Biopolitics in the Pharmacopornographic Era.* Translated by Bruce Benderson. The Feminist Press, 2013.

Prokhoris, Sabine. *L'Insaisissable Histoire de la Psychanalyse.* Presses Universitaires de France, 2014.

Roth-Bettoni, Didier. *L'Homosexualité au cinema.* Paris, La Musardine, 2007.

Rubin, Gayle. "The Traffic in Women: Notes on the Political Economy of Sex." In *Toward an Anthropology of Women.* Edited by Rayna R. Reiter. Monthly Review Press, 1975.

Sastre, Peggy. *No Sex. Avoir envie de ne pas faire l'amour.* La Musardine, 2010.

Sedgwick, Eve Kosofsky. *Epistemology of the Closet.* University of California Press, 1990.

Voros, Florian (ed.). *Cultures pornographiques.* Anthologie des Porn studies. Editions Amsterdam, 2015.

Wittig, Monique. "The Straight Mind." In *The Straight Mind and Other Essays.* Beacon Press, 1992.

Chapter 2

The Ruins of Oedipus

Oedipus in a major key

With regular frequency, and quite recently even, a number of psychoanalysts – thankfully not all[1] – have taken turns appearing in various media outlets in order to mourn the disappearance of the well-known Oedipus complex, drawing a stark picture of the irremediable risks that this entails for civilization as a whole. On each and every occasion, such statements reinforce the four-poled structure deplored by the queer movement. In other words, a great number of Freud's heirs continue to declare their indefectible allegiance to the Oedipal law. In this, they set forth their attachment to the traditional family structure of father, mother, child, warning against any alternatives. At the same time, they foreground their solid belief in a structure and a line of thought that we would have difficulty in qualifying, together with the novelist and postfeminist theorist Monique Wittig, as anything other than "straight" (read as "normal," "regular," "square," and "heterosexual"). The attachment to the Oedipus complex, in its most stale conception in any case, is the veritable cornerstone of this line of thought which operates in a major key: secure in its universality, established by white heterosexual men, this notion dominates and imposes its patterns of thought upon all forms of alterity. Reading queer theory relativizes the validity of the Oedipal reference as the sole civilizational template. Sailing beyond Oedipus, and moving past its siren-song, doubtlessly constitutes the first horizon to which a clinic in a minor key aspires. But before exploring these foreign shores, let us rapidly remember precisely what the Oedipal tragedy consists of as it rings out within psychoanalysis in a major key.

In a letter to his friend Fliess, the father of psychoanalysis mentions, for the first time, the germ of this idea which would later became a general principle:

> I have found, in my own case too, falling in love with the mother and jealousy of the father, and I now regard it as a universal event of early childhood [...]. If that is so, we can understand the riveting power of

DOI: 10.4324/9781003612735-2

> *Oedipus Rex*, in spite of all the objections raised by reason against its presupposition of destiny.[2]

Building on this missive, Freud unceasingly returned to this idea which he continuously elaborated, charting the ramifications of the notion down to the smallest detail. The essential structure was however already in place: within *himself* Freud discovered the universality of love felt towards the mother and jealousy towards the father. He immediately drew a parallel between this discovery and the Greek tragedy. More than a hundred years later the famous Oedipus complex remains, far too often, one of the principal and foundational notions of psychoanalysis within the collective imagination.

Is it even necessary to repeat the hackneyed chapter and verse? Have Freud's successors not repeated, with nauseating frequency, the phrases that rhythm the *normal* development of the libido?

The trajectory of this development follows a straight line from the oral stage (where the privileged zone of gratification corresponds to the mouth, as explored through breastfeeding and thumb sucking), traverses the anal stage (through bowel control), arriving at the phallic stage (with a corresponding interest in the genital erogenous zone). At this juncture, the Oedipal tragedy is ineluctably bound to play out as the child is seen as obliged to fall in love with the parent of the opposite sex and confront their rivalry in the parent of the same sex. As everyone knows, before reaching the relative peace of the latent phase, the youth would have to tackle the equally well-known and disturbing inverse side of the Oedipal drama: the castration complex.

A number of difficulties arise out of this version of Freud's theory. This is particularly true as concerns women: why does the young girl no longer love her mother, and why does she fear castration given that she does not possess a penis? If the experience of the phallic stage is limited to that of young boys, the corresponding relations become substantially easier for young girls. As Herman Nunberg, the imperturbable post-Freudian reminds us, summarizing the Freudian Oedipal position:

> It is not quite clear how it happens that there is identification at one time with the parent of the same sex, at another time with the parent of the opposite sex. It is assumed that a constitutional factor forms the biological basis for bisexuality, at one time exerting pressure toward identification in the direction of the masculine, at another time of the feminine strivings.[3]

This schema, while plausible for the young boy, plunged Freud himself into insurmountable difficulties when it came to the question of young girls. How are we to understand the Oedipal turning point when the young girl desires her father and her mother becomes a hateful object, and how to introduce the presence of the feminine superego?

Bisexuality and penis envy in young girls (*Penisneid*) have both been raised by Freud in order to better understand this "dark continent"[4] of femininity. And if it was, in a word, quite audacious to envisage bisexuality in all human beings, this discovery was rejected with equally rapid aplomb. On one hand, it is useful only in so far as it aids in overcoming the difficulties linked to the expression of feminine sexuality during the phallic stage, on the other, it does not amount to an expression of the indecisive nature of sexuality. Rather it acts, by and large, to confirm the distribution of masculine and feminine roles and the normal separation of activity and passivity that is derived therefrom.

This reminder of the Oedipal gospel illustrates the degree to which a traditionalist representation, to say the least, of life and of sexual conduct can be drawn from Freud's writings. "The masculine aim is active; the feminine aim is passive. Activity or passivity thus also is determined by the anatomical structure of the reproductive organs."[5] Ultimately Freud himself, and of his own accord, admitted that he was not convinced by the torturous logic of his solution.

It is clear that nothing works in Freud's writing. He vainly attempts to establish a line of symmetry between the sexes: castration anxiety on the masculine side and penis envy (*Penisneid*) on the feminine side. He is forced to introduce the young girl into the Oedipal at the very moment when the young boy escapes from it. In other words, if the young boy resolves to abandon his mother as an exclusive object of love when faced with the father's threat of castration, the young girl enters into the Oedipal conflict upon realization of her castration and calls on her father in order to obtain the phallus. Given what we have just illustrated, feminist and postfeminist thought has every reason to be outraged.

Wittig's rage

Gender theories, in their efforts to separate sex, grounded in biology, from gender, culturally constructed, and even to demonstrate how the representation of the binarity of the sexes is itself a result of cultural constructions, is thus opposed to the classical vision of *the* difference between the sexes as expressed in Freud and by the Oedipus complex.[6] In fact, all of the correlates which have been culturally acquired and which flow forth from the Oedipal scenario (passivity, activity, femininity, masculinity, heterosexuality, homosexuality, and so on) wind up being reduced to biology and flounder on the shores of purported natural dispositions. However, there is worse to come. The Oedipal scenario is not satisfied in merely being a powerful staging post for the fixation of sexuality, of bodies, and for channelling the libidinal fluxes of successive psychodevelopmental stages. The Oedipal scenario encodes. It structures. It frames the very manner in which we relate to ourselves.[7] In speaking the language of Oedipus we are always at risk of losing the plurality of languages at work in the worldly Real. To exclusively follow its laws is to follow but a single of the "signifying highways."[8] This trap snaps shut once we begin to believe that there is but one way of thinking, speaking, and loving. That which is *straight*.

Without a doubt, Wittig never intended to think in an orthodox manner. She accepted neither well-meaning self-evidences, nor a straight and narrow interpretation. Even of that which ensures the general uptake of the normative consensus. She rejected language with its forceful grammatical certitudes where, in French, as in too many other languages, in an almost symptomatic fashion, the masculine takes precedence over the feminine. Wittig laid her cards on the table, confronting "straight thought" in a scathing manner. She quite literally and visually shattered language itself.[9] Her rage was well founded. It reflected the violence suffered.

According to Wittig, women submit themselves to men, first and foremost within heterosexual relationships. Everything contributes to the reproduction of this form of relationship. As highlighted by structuralism, the reign of the symbolic, with the key roles played by the phallus and the Oedipus complex, would, drawing on "very few elements,"[10] definitively result in this mechanic. The system of exchange propagated by the symbolic order[11] not only ensures the reproduction of the species, but has taken root within our language, our ideas, our representations, our concepts and even the manner in which we articulate them. This engenders the creation of "a society where heterosexuality would not order not only all human relationships but also its very production of concepts and all the processes which escape consciousness, as well."[12] A straight vision of society is silently imposed at every turn of phrase, in the unspoken moral of each and every concept, in the secret longings of every proposition.

The theoretician asks herself:

> What is this thought which refuses to reverse itself, which never puts into question what primarily constitutes it? This thought is the dominant thought. It is a thought which affirms an "already there" of the sexes, something which is supposed to have come before all thought, before all society. This thought is the thought of those who rule over women.[13]

Wittig pertinently points out the blatant allure of some forms of reasoning, in so far as their interrogation is of little use to the dominant majority. But, as soon as anyone launches into a careful reconsideration of these certitudes, they quite suddenly shatter. One could say that *straight* thought constitutes the *a priori*, a framework which is not in and of itself called into question, but within which all interrogations are inscribed. Wittig thus shifts (hetero-)sexual difference from its position as a biological marker of distinction, to the political domain.

To what degree does psychoanalytic thought, constructed in Oedipal terms, despite its use of free association, despite its openness to the discoveries of the unconscious, and despite echoing the trajectory of the drives, contribute to the erection of a paradigm of *straight* thought? Is the psychoanalytic unconscious strictly locked into the domain of *straight* thought? And were it to escape, could we specify how?

For Wittig the struggle and the debate are essentially over. She asserts:

> Our refusal of the totalizing interpretation of psychoanalysis makes the theoreticians say that we neglect the symbolic dimension. [...] These discourses speak about us and claim to say the truth in an apolitical field, as if anything of that which signifies could escape the political in this moment of history, and as if, in what concerns us, politically insignificant signs could exist.[14]

The position of women, more precisely that of lesbians, can no longer abide the machinations of psychoanalytical interpretation. Of course, the primary adversary, here, is the phallic signifier.[15] Further on in her deconstruction of the self-evident silence of the anatomical politics of language, Wittig clarifies that:

> Thus one speaks of *the* exchange of women, *the* difference between the sexes, *the* symbolic order, *the* Unconscious, Desire, *Jouissance*, Culture, History, giving an absolute meaning to these concepts when they are only categories founded upon heterosexuality, or thought which produces the difference between the sexes as a political and philosophical dogma.[16]

Women themselves are not spared from Wittig's rage. In following, letter by letter, her logic of unwriting the phallogocentric order, she forsakes her own position as a woman, adopting that of a lesbian and reconstructing a body and corpus through writing,[17] going so far as to reassess the very notion of a dictionary,[18] reinventing language through poetry. Wittig's project is ambitious, utopian even. She sought to eradicate any reference to the matrix through which the world is rendered intelligible and to which psychoanalysis subscribes. Indeed, this matrix is weighed down with inequalities, incapable of taking the plurality of differences into account in so far as it foregrounds only one difference: that between men and women.[19] Yet, to speak of *the* necessary, universal, absolute, incommensurable, inevitable difference between the sexes, is, quite often, to valorize, or even legitimize, one form of sexuality where one sex completes the other, to the detriment of marginal sexualities. The latter turn of phrase is to be understood as including the numerous forms of relationship where dual or binary opposition seems, simply, to be less important, or which are structured in terms other than those of heterosexuality.[20] According to Wittig, lesbians, as the primary victims of this system of domination, cannot, under any circumstances, come to terms with being identified by way of a category that is conceived of in their stead by an oppressor. Hence her phrase: "Lesbians are not women."[21]

Wittig has however not refused to take the unconscious into consideration. Its importance propelled her to include it in her *Dictionary*: "Warning to the companion lovers, if you have an unconscious, you know all about it. But if you have one all the more reason to be careful of the traffickers of the unconscious."[22] So as to guard against the traffickers, both male and female, of the unconscious Wittig seems to opt for, in parenthesis, the reading of the unconscious offered by Deleuze and Guattari:

> For us there are, it seems, not one or two sexes but many (cf. Guattari/ Deleuze), as many sexes as there are individuals. [...] Sexuality is for us an inevitable battleground insofar as we want to get outside of genitality and of the sexual economy imposed on us by the dominant heterosexuality.[23]

Wittig's anger with regard to the dominant heterosexuality explicitly joins that of Deleuze and Guattari concerning the Oedipus complex. In fact, she depends upon it. We shall at once take the measure of the importance of this parenthesis.

Introduction to *Anti-Oedipus*

In considering the work of Deleuze and Guattari, we are able to at once take a closer look at both psychoanalysis and queer theory. Wittig's furtive call to Deleuze and Guattari's *n* sexes thus merits further development.

From 1972, in *Anti-Oedipus*, and in the wake of the sexual revolution of May 1968, Gilles Deleuze and Félix Guattari launched a violent crusade against psychoanalysis. Their goal was none other than to establish an understanding of the unconscious that was no longer radically normalized by the Oedipal scenario. They sought to establish a "schizoanalysis."

The two authors did thus not dismiss the unconscious. They renewed the approach. They did not fall prey to the trap of a "thinking though," but on the contrary, remained in constant contact with the abyss unlocked by the unconscious. According to them, language in a major key as expressed in Freudian psychoanalysis was insufficient when it came to uncovering the realm of dreams and of madness. The norms determined by those in power could not take account of the wealth of the unconscious.

Anti-Oedipus, virulent firebrand targeting the field of analysis regulated by the Oedipal figure, is, in fact, a formidable love song for the unconscious. In retrospect, both the anger levelled against psychoanalytic interpretation, and the radical destabilisation of identity, extolled by this work found a home at the heart of certain queer critiques.[24] Deleuze and Guattari characterized their work as a "collective arrangement of enunciation."[25] Through the use of this concept they refused to assign a given thought to a given subject, to a given author. For them there was no enunciative subject, no intellectual property, no copyright. They preferred to advocate for the fluxes and multiplicities which inhabit us on an unconscious level, and which force us into becoming something other than merely an Ego. Subjectivity was thus left bleeding. And liberation from the Oedipal yoke partook in the discovery of impersonal individuations.

In their works, their condemnation of the Oedipal is without appeal: "each time the subject strikes up the song of myth or intones tragic lines, carrying him back *to the factory*."[26] The principal rebuke addressed at psychoanalysis is that it is a motor for the creation of the Oedipal. That is to say that psychoanalysis forces subjects, through the cure, into a triangularization of their desire, affixing their desire to a compliant subject. Deleuze and Guattari sought to invert this manner of relating to the unconscious, taking hold of the unconscious in a resolutely non-theatrical manner. Their approach to desire is thus in terms of mechanics and production. They thereby turn their backs on the diminutive theatrics of the Oedipal triangle as represented by "daddy-mommy-me."[27]

The diminutive Oedipal theatre

Let us once again remind ourselves of several self-evident truths before moving further long with the work of Deleuze and Guattari. In quoting Fechner, Freud defined the "special particularities of dream-life" as a different "scene of action."[28] He affirms that "the scene of action of dreams is different from that of waking ideational life."[29] Two scenes are contrasted here: that of the diurnal self and that of the unconscious. Other than this definition of the dream-life and the sphere of the unconscious as a scene, the ties that bind psychoanalysis to theatre are numerous. The most familiar, the most oft cited, is that of the cruel tragedy that we all know so well. "What I have in mind is the legend of King Oedipus and Sophocles' drama which bears his name"[30] whose "profound and universal power to move can only be understood if the hypothesis I have put forward in regard to the psychology of children has an equally universal validity."[31] It is the "validity" of this diminutive Oedipal theatre, its "universal power," which are drawn from a "hypothesis" that the theories of gender deconstruction question. In truth, strictly read from the point of view of the Oedipus complex, the *talking cure* winds up taking on well-worn moralizing tones.

The analytic apparatus, governed by the "profound and universal power"[32] of the Oedipal law, would impose a structural law on humankind. It would, therefore, be irremediably tarnished by, at the very least, a heteronormative, or even a homophobic dimension. Heteronormative insofar as the position of desire, that of a mature and authentic desire, would correspond to that of a heterosexual subject. Homophobic insofar as homosexuality, thus considered, is an anomaly, a failure in the development of the subject, or at best, a form of arrested development.

We thus understand the utility and the necessity of the cumbersome proceedings against psychoanalysis undertaken by Deleuze and Guattari. They go so far as to encompass what seems like destruction. "Destroy, destroy. The task of schizoanalysis goes by way of destruction – a whole scoring of the unconscious, a complete cutterage. Destroy Oedipus, the illusion of the ego, the puppet of the superego, guilt, the law, castration."[33] Seeking to allow for the advent of desire without reference to the subject, melts away more than one aspect of the Freudian iceberg. Of course, the authors remind us: "If someone reading this book feels that things are fine in psychoanalysis, we're not speaking for him, and for him we take back everything we have said."[34]

Machinic desire and desiring micropolitics

Anti-Oedipus opens with a highly colourful homage to Judge Schreber: "Judge Schreber has sunbeams in his ass. *A solar anus.* And rest assured that it works: Judge Schreber feels something, produces something and is capable of explaining the process theoretically. Something is produced: the effects of a machine, not mere metaphors."[35]

From the very first lines of their volume, thanks to the character of Judge Schreber, Deleuze and Guattari lay out their path, composed almost entirely of warnings against that which they deem to be analytical shortcuts. The character of Judge Schreber plunges our thoughts directly into the sexual. And this, more than merely making sense, has something to do with production. It is only from the point of view of this sexual production that a theory can be sketched out, and not inversely. They do not seek to tame the sexual through a turn of phrase, to frame the real by way of metaphor, through meaningful impressions, but, on the contrary, they seek to embrace the physical dimension of the connections that emerge out of the memories of the famous judge, president of an appeals court in Dresden.

Herein lies one of the points of contention with regards to the analytic orthodoxy: there is nothing missing in desire. It is constituted by fluxes, branches, connections. All of these elements order themselves and extend far beyond the subject. The latter becoming, in effect, a hub of machinic connections. Thus, the coordinates that shape us are no longer exclusively private, intimate, familial, but are dependent upon the social, the economic, and the technological. One does not desire in the same way in a given place, at a given time, or in terms of such and such a technology.

> The unconscious is totally unaware of persons as such. Partial objects are not representations of parental figures or of the basic patterns of family relations; they are parts of desiring-machines, having to do with a

> process and with relations of production that are both irreducible and prior to anything that may be made to conform to the Oedipal figure.[36]

In a word, desire is machinic.

Based on this, the authors propose a "desiring micropolitics." This complicated notion is not so much attached to the determination of the stakes of power where it is explicitly exercised (in a "molar" manner, to use their terms), but rather to the miniscule movements that escape perception, and which nevertheless traverse our lives. These imperceptible movements, "molecular," can incessantly cause us to shift: either they plunge us into rigid, binary, and fatal thoughts – thoughts of judgement; or, on the contrary, they open us to new becomings, unexpected and infinite – asubjective desires.[37] For Deleuze and Guattari desire is always desire of desire. Here again, their dissent from a psychoanalytic reading could not be more pronounced. Let us remember that, for Lacan rereading Freud, desire is nothing more than lack. In this, psychoanalysis no doubt participates in a classical philosophical tradition that Deleuze and Guattari chose to abandon. We must however insist upon their relative ambiguity regarding the teachings of Lacan: they are as critical as they are respectful. In point of fact, Lacan, and this is at the heart of his significance from a minor point of view, does not advance *Anti-Oedipus* so much as he goes beyond it.

Whatever the case may be, according to Deleuze and Guattari, even structuralist illuminations which foregrounded Oedipus from a signifying point of view, remain instrumental in the normalization of the unconscious. Plotting out the signifier continues to provide analysis with inescapable laws. If we do not call into question the force with which these laws are imposed, we are blinded to the relation between psychoanalysis and power. Nevertheless, Deleuze and Guattari perfectly illustrated the fact that they had heard the phrase in which Lacan distanced himself from the Freudian Oedipus. They write:

> Here too Lacan's approach appears in all its complexity; for it is certain that he does not enclose the unconscious in an Oedipal structure. He shows, on the contrary that Oedipus is imaginary, nothing but an image, a myth; that this or these images are produced by an oedipalizing structure, that this structure acts only insofar as it reproduces the element of castration which itself is not imaginary but symbolic.[38]

In short order I'll come back to the complexity and the importance of this undertaking and on the manner in which we can draw on this to construe, not an anti-Oedipal clinic, as Deleuze and Guattari would have liked, but rather one that is well and truly post-Oedipal.

For the time being, let us remark that, for our two authors, Lacan seems to

> Maintain a kind of projection of the signifying chains onto a despotic signifier, lacking unto itself and reintroducing the lack into a series of desire on which it imposed an exclusive use. Was it possible to denounce Oedipus-as-myth, and nevertheless maintain that the castration complex itself was not a myth but in fact something real?[39]

If Deleuze and Guattari would have liked to definitively rid themselves of Oedipus in advocating for a schizoanalysis, it is certainly not so as to value the return of the phallus as the only signifier which escapes either signification or castration.

Upon writing *Anti-Oedipus*, Deleuze and Guattari are quite clear: they refuse both a conceptualization of desire as being intertwined with the notion of lack, and they refuse any conceptualization of the unconscious with reference, even symbolically, to castration. Another type of bond with the unconscious must be uncovered: one that at last liberates from judgement, one that releases delirium from its neurotic or psychotic impasses and reconciles it with desire:

> Delirium is a disease, the disease par excellence, whenever it erects a race it claims is pure and dominant. But it is the measure of health when it invokes this oppressed bastard race that ceaselessly stirs beneath dominations, resisting everything that crushes and imprisons, a race that is outlined in relief in literature as process.[40]

The authors of *Anti-Oedipus* thus abandoned an interpretation of delirium charted in terms of the family so as to understand what it signified. Rather, they strive to understand *how it works*. The question is not "what does *it* mean?" but "how does *it* work?" What matters to them is to appreciate how delirium relates to "history, race, continents." They thus place a social mechanism in opposition to the significatory mechanism of psychoanalysis. In affirming that the unconscious is machinic we can think of it as being beyond its strictly linguistic treatment. We dig ourselves out from beneath the sole reference to the phallic guide. Thus, when they analyse the delirium of judge Schreber, Deleuze and Guattari are not as attached to the pathological manifestations as they are to the social mechanisms of the malady. This is a response to the dysfunctions of capitalism. "Every delirium is first of all the investment of a field that is social, economic, political, cultural, racial and racist, pedagogical, and religious: the delirious person applies a delirium to his family and his son that overreaches them on all sides."[41]

This is what the father of psychoanalysis did not want to understand. Instead of leaving the field of play open to libidinal productions, instead of stimulating the simulacra of subjective essence, Freud would have preferred to anchor them to the representations of the Ego with the Oedipal law as intermediary. This is another manner of translating the famous Freudian statement "Wo es war, soll Ich werden."[42] Thus armed with the language of the Oedipal law and his inherent familism, the psychoanalyst would weigh the capacity (or incapacity) of the Ego to find its way within its meagre perimeter enclosed by neurosis or psychosis. In so doing, he would miss out on the possibility of experiencing the multiplicities characteristic of unconscious productions. If Oedipus constitutes a prerequisite that determines the "normality" of the subject, it thereby gives birth to a binary territory that banishes that which does not conform to its representation: the powers (*puissances*), the multiplicities, the affects, the percepts which can never directly be attributed to the unity of an Ego. Again, in other words, with Oedipus – conceived as the law by which man is bound to language, as the mark of language upon the body[43] – Freud gave a human and acceptable face to a libido which, in reality, would be machinic, delirious, desiring, composed of incessant fluxes. Freud could have drawn open the curtains, revealing the universal molecular forces that animate us and risk, in every moment, overwhelming us, causing us to stammer, become delirious, and desire by other means: no longer in the shadow of death and guilt. Taking Oedipus as the unavoidable point of departure for the cure and considering it as an imaginary reflection of familial norms is tantamount to either ignoring, foreclosing, or even condemning parental, relational, desiring configurations that cannot be squared with the sacrosanct model. This can also be expressed in the terms employed by Gayle Rubin, the queer anthropologist that we referenced earlier: "in the most general terms, the Oedipal complex is a machine which fashions the appropriate forms of sexual individuals."[44] In their own way queer communities have taken up the torch of Deleuze and Guattari in disassembling this machine so as to invent others. The reflections on the body and on power as they have been expressed since the AIDS crisis assert the importance of

> nonfigurative loves, indices of a revolutionary investment of the social field, and which are neither Oedipal nor pre-oedipal since it all amounts to the same thing, but innocently anoedipal [...]. Undoing the form of persons and the ego, not in behalf of a pre-oedipal undifferentiated, but in behalf of anoedipal lines of singularities, the desiring-machines.[45]

Becoming and *n* sexes

The anti-Oedipal virulence takes on its full meaning when, in *A Thousand Plateaus*, the second volume of their collective work, Deleuze and Guattari consider the question of becoming-minor. For them the minorities, more than being, have to escape being, to actualize becomings, to defy fixed identities, to create lines of flight outside of any preestablished trajectories, to race off at hitherto unthinkable speeds. The inhabitants of these margins, those who do not identify themselves as possessing power, those who have difficulty tolerating the white-masculine-heterosexual-petty-bourgeois majority, those who do not succeed in settling beneath the banner of Oedipal logic, have to affirm their desire in a molecular manner, to put the majoritarian system and its personal, egoic norms, and its inevitable violence to flight. In no instance can they continue to be within what they are.

A micropolitical reconquest of the libido abandons the anthropological representation of sex. The latter is the principal relay of an oppressive dispositive, that of the language of power, sole formulation of our existence in a major key. Put to service an anonymous standard, such a representation is incapable of understanding (or hearing even) the demands and capacities which would revolutionize our being, at work in all of those who are without a voice, in all of those who have been condemned to silence. In fact, those who hold power have no interest in hearing those who speak, articulate, formulate their existence in any way other than with Oedipus as the starting block.

In discovering desiring-machines which, a far cry from the Oedipal, throb and hum, we reconnect with the revolutionary power of the unconscious. We thus set off toward becomings that break through, that flee, that escape the restricted domain of the Ego, the individual and the subject. In this way, and in opposition to fixed identities, Deleuze and Guattari foster becoming-women, becoming-black, becoming-homosexual. Their theory of becoming incites us to take a closer and more critical look at the masculine/feminine opposition, to deconstruct our sex and our gender identity. Contemplate *n* sexes rather than two, in a strictly anthropological representation.

The sexuality that matters to them is nonhuman. It is neither animal nor savage but refers to libidinal investment and the manner in which this is organized within the social field. "The truth is that sexuality is everywhere: the way a bureaucrat fondles his records, a judge administers justice, a businessman causes money to circulate; the bourgeoisie fucks the proletariat and so on."[46] In other words, for them, sexuality must be released from the complete image of Man. In each and every moment, sexuality can transform itself, discerning not merely two sexes but *n* sexes. "If sexuality is the unconscious investment of the large molar aggregates, it is because on its other side sexuality is identical with the interplay of the molecular elements that constitute these aggregates under determined conditions."[47] Thus, the possibility, nay the necessity for each and everyone, delirious or not, to not become a Man but to engage in a becoming-woman. Therein too lies the necessity, not only to ask what a woman is, but how to become one? So, the question is no longer "are you a man or a woman?" but rather "where do you situate yourself, in which domain?" "How does your jouissance work, what are the gears of your desiring-machines?" This amounts to the disappearance of one, and one single sex, so that the swarming multiplicities of the sexual domain may arise. Schreber himself may have passed over into the domain of becoming, escaping his paranoid molar configuration by becoming the wife of god.

> The love blockage [...] curiously changes its function, depending on whether it engages desire in the Oedipal impasses of the couple and the family in the service of the repressive machines, or whether on the contrary it condenses a free energy capable of fuelling a revolutionary machine.[48]

As we can see, desire and delirium are two forms of the libido that adjoin so as to defy any notion of sexual identity as fixed and frozen.

In this sense, Deleuze and Guattari's theorization allows for a glimpse of a becoming-woman of woman, a becoming-woman of man, a molecular multiplicity at work beneath the surface of every one of us: "Desiring-machines or the nonhuman sex: not one or even two sexes, but *n* sexes."[49]

The theorization of Deleuze and Guattari culminates in a reformulation of the body, in its liberation, in its perpetual transformation: *ad litteram*, in their view, we will never have finished becoming something other than ourselves. We will never cease our transformation by means of unconscious, virtual and molecular fluxes. These fluxes encircle us and, once we encounter them, they prevent the actualization of our dominant beings and majoritarian identities. This agenda proves to be quite delightful. In any case, it worked its charms on Wittig. *Out* with the identitarian body and its binary oppositions of man/woman, homosexual/heterosexual, active/passive, heart/mind. What is revealed is the construction of a body without organs, a body without organicity: being between, leaving figuration behind, differentiating beyond, or short of, the binary.

Moving beyond Oedipus

Presently, we better understand to what degree Deleuze and Guattari's break with the Oedipal unconscious intersects with Wittig's questions. In both instances the ferocity of the anti-Oedipal case is without limits. In this context, were we to approach the unconscious from a theatrical standpoint, this could only be undertaken in following Artaud's Theatre of Cruelty. The fluxes, the shit and the screams thrust us far beyond ourselves, far from any neurotic subject. Collapse of the Ego, forsaking language, the possibility of hallucinatory conceptions from other worlds is ever present. "Overturn the theatre of representation into the order of desiring-production: this is the whole task of schizoanalysis."[50] Such desiring-machines are as fascinating as they are schizoid.

On a daily basis, the clinician encounters the unbearable: that which hobbles each of us in our existence, that which unceasingly provokes suffering, that which is unable to go back to normal. The handbook of the anti-Oedipal workshop is not always easy to comprehend. When faced with the subject's complaint, how does one make use of it? Hearing the machinic humming, lending an ear to the grumbling deliriums shot through with the hallucinations of race, history, continents, and languages, all sharpen clinical attentiveness. Reading *Anti-Oedipus* propels the analytic goodwill and its evenly suspended attention into the Beyond. It awakens the vigilance of the therapist. When faced with minorities – gays, lesbians, blacks, trans, bi, *queers* … – at times stigmatized, at times fascinated by the capitalist potencies and the innumerable possibilities that the latter offer the body, what does the cure propose? What social, ethical trajectories, what words and which actions does it marshal? What forms of hope and possibility does it open up for those who, sometimes obliged or forced, undertake this experience? In other words, how, and in what way is the clinic always already political?

Anti-Oedipal thought, following that of Wittig, calls for an alternative to the Oedipal mythology. Is this an effective solution? It sweeps the Sophoclean tragedy away, together with its adherent series of binarisms. It gives way to an imaginary so surprising, so revolutionary and so powerful that we may even be tempted to question its efficacity in the context of the modest quotidian of the cure. For their part, the perspectives foregrounded by queer theory also call the Oedipal postulate into question. Nevertheless, the ideal of a "society without gender," more than a radical move away from the Oedipal myth, is rather, and without doubt, borne out of an internal deconstruction. Queer theories, in their own way, sketch the contours of a passage not to the anti-Oedipal, but to the post-Oedipal. In a way this movement connects with what we could call, in anticipation of the advances that Lacan proposes in his final teachings, a clinic of jouissance, of case-by-case *nouage.* [51]

The notion of a logic where the Oedipal no longer corresponds to the first reliable reference or is the sole analysis necessary for the constitution of the subject requires setting out to strenuously trace the concours of new cartographies, capable of welcoming post-Oedipal subjectivities. The latter shake up familiar certitudes. They question the very foundation of the intelligibility of the world of the psyche. Even though they offer new contours regarding chosen relations (in terms of love, family, and communities etc.) they do not, however, escape the stakes of repression which are specific to the unconscious. A clinic in a minor key thus sets itself the task of inventing new ways of hearing the subject's complaint, of mapping out their subjectivities.[52] This also means questioning anew the manner in which the drive is stressed in discourse, regardless of the novelty of its contours. It means envisaging the Oedipal, not as universal, but rather as a possible manner, at a given time, in which subjectivity may have been constituted. What remains is to pinpoint, among the ruins of the Oedipal, how contemporary subjects set about living, suffering, and loving.

Lacan and the law of language

From another point of view, moving beyond the Oedipal could also be the point of the position developed by Lacan in the course of his teachings.

When, to begin with, he takes up the Oedipal, far from any conception centred on maturity or the childhood development of the Ego, he articulates it in accordance with a logic that is sketched out over a period of time. In his understanding, father, mother, and child are nothing more than positions which determine the manner in which human beings are integrated into language. The paternal function plays a determinant role in so far as it makes isolation, the disjunction between the child and the child's desire for the mother, possible: the father drives the mother to a back and forth between him and the child. She seems thus to desire something other than the child: the mother desires the phallus of which the father is the bearer.

The famous Lacanian aphorism "the unconscious is structured like a language" condenses this structuration of desire by the Oedipal and the phallus. For as long as the child has not encountered the paternal metaphor, the child remains an indeterminate subject, subject to the uncontrolled law of the mother. For the child, the substitution of the Name-of-the-Father for the desire of the mother provokes a change in register: the emergence of phallic signification. Such is the classical version of the Lacanian Oedipus: the interplay of positions wherein desire is inscribed into its intimate relationship with language. A symbolic strategy relieved of the weight of the body, of the concrete reality of character, and attached to the interplay of signifiers is implemented. In other words, Oedipus becomes guarantor of access to the symbolic order: "In the rule of the Name-of-the-Father, he [the child] steps out of indetermination and is inscribed with a precise signification, the phallic signification which corresponds to that which the paternal signifier produces upon the child."[53] We can, however, read this account of the subject's accession to language in a major key, in reifying the positions and roles in absolute terms, as indisputable ontological conditions rigorously ascribed to the heterosexual trinity of daddy-mommy-child.

On the contrary, in a minor key, we could consider that the father only plays the role of a metaphor and that he does not personify the phallus: he is merely the symbol thereof. The father is not the phallus but rather represents the person who has the phallus in so far as this figure can fill the maternal lack. As Lacan explains in his seminar:

> the Name-of-the-Father has the function of signifying the entire system of signifiers, authorizing its existence, making it law [...] the phallus enters into play in the signifying system when the subject has to symbolize [...] the signified as such, [...] what he desires. [...] The phallus is the signifier of the signified in general.[54]

This affirmation cuts against the grain of Freud's proposition in *Analysis Terminable and Interminable* and revitalises it, pushing it in a new direction: the other side that an analysis can never reach is not a question of fear for the loss of the penis, or the desire thereof, but rather the complete understanding of the phallus as signifier of desire. At this juncture, we can ask ourselves: do the laws of the signifier, conceived of in terms of spaces and structures, reproduce the peculiarities of a sexuality strictly formulated in heteronormative terms or can they open up to new familial configurations?

In any case, the transition towards a symbolic register has substantial consequences for the psychoanalytic clinic. Analysis no longer sees itself as an instrument of healing, if by healing we understand a definitive identification or a closure of the inherent scission wrought by the mark of language. The phallus "can play its role only when veiled, that is, as itself a sign of the latency with which any signifiable is struck, once it is raised (*aufgehoben*) to the function of the signifier. The phallus is the signifier of this very *Aufhebung*, which it inaugurates (initiates) by its disappearance."[55] More precisely, the phallus, envisioned through the regime of the signifier, refers to an evanescence which coincides with that of desire: as signifier of signifiers the phallus can never be rendered consistent and only appears as veiled, repressed. "It is only conceivable if it has already implied that it is the signifier of lack, the signifier of the distance between the subject's demand and his desire."[56]

What takes place is the economy of the unconscious which thus reveals the subject's dependence upon language. This bond will determine, for each and every one, the modalities of their desire, their jouissance, in short, their relationship with the world. The substitution of the Name-of-the-Father for the desire of the mother, that is to say the paternal metaphor, shackles the subject to the yoke of the law of the signifier. More simply, we can say that the transition through the Oedipus complex and its reverse side, the castration complex, results in a conception of language as castration and of desire as lack. Certainly, this is the key aspect of the turnaround that Freud undergoes when read through Lacanian structuralism: linguistic castration implies a conception of desire as lack. The phallus is thus the fundamental signifier through which man's desire and that of woman attempt to be acknowledged by each other.

Lacan does however concede that the remainder of the formulations relating to the formation of sexual identity retain a normalizing aspect. "The Oedipus complex has an essential normalizing function."[57] As he states further on, "It is, in other words, about my showing you from what perspective, from what approach we get an insight into the possibility of normativization – therapeutic normativization."[58] Or even: "the Oedipus complex has a normative function, not simply in the subject's moral structure, or in his relations with reality, but concerning the assumption of his sex, which, as you know, still retains a certain ambiguity in analysis."[59]

It is upon this ambiguity that Judith Butler founds her radical deconstruction of potentially homophobic, heteronormative, and binary preconceptions within psychoanalysis. In understanding the stakes, both ironic and political, of this deconstruction, we do not give up on analysis as a practice. Nor, by the same measure, do we adhere to an anti-Oedipal ideal. On the contrary, we will perhaps be able to cross paths with novel nuances in the analytic field: not merely from a metaphyschological point of view, but also from a clinical perspective.

Judith Butler and gender

Judith Butler addresses subalterns, those unrecognized, those constrained to silence. She articulates her thought in taking as her point of departure the violence that the oppressed experience within their own bodies. Her thought plots and weaves through the suffering of one and all. As a feminist, her thinking took its initial starting point in the difficulty that one may have in identifying oneself with one's own gender, regardless of one's sex. There are, in her opinion, presuppositions, linguistic norms, attitudes which hinder, or even foreclose, any consideration of lives that do not feel that they are in alignment with the binary division of sex and their social representation which articulates two, and only two, genders.

> Gender is a complexity whose totality is permanently deferred, never fully what it is at any given juncture in time. An open coalition, then, will affirm identities that are alternately instituted and relinquished according to the purposes at hand; it will be an open assemblage that permits of multiple convergences and divergences without obedience to a normative telos of definitional closure.[60]

Butler thus uses gender to disqualify any rigidification of our being and our lives ("a man reacts like this," "a woman surely enjoys herself like that"). The explicit finality of her philosophy is to extend the spectrum of possibilities "so that we might actually have a broader conception of how human beings do make meaning in their lives and what gives their lives meaning."[61] Faced with the anxiety that those who are outside the norm experience, and confronted by the same emotion that they inspire in those who inhabit the world in a major key, gender is a tool that can be used to understand the difficulties that both groups feel. Mapping out the consequences of these difficulties leads to nothing other than a crisis within well-established divisions. In her preface to the 1999 edition of *Gender Trouble*, Butler explains: "This doesn't mean that all minority practices are to be condoned or celebrated, but it does mean that we ought to be able to think them before we come to any kinds of conclusions about them."[62] Disrupting the preconception of the binary is not an easy task.

Despite the solidity of its appearance, the problematization of gender uncovers its profound precarity, its intrinsic vulnerability, and its extreme variability. Taking cognizance thereof engenders an ontological crisis that could lead to new capacities for thinking with those excluded from majoritarian grammar: giving them a voice with which to express the logic of the world and the universal in an alternate manner.

Butler affirms: "our notions of what a human being [...is...] problematically depend on there being two coherent genders. And if someone doesn't comply with either the masculine norm or the feminine norm, their very humanness is called into question."[63] Her work relativizes thus the scope of both *difference* and of *sex*. We will come back to this. For the moment, let us consider how philosophy manages to reflect the Oedipal structure in a minor key.

Butler as a reader of Lacan

The work of psychoanalysis in a minor key is to investigate the domain of the drives without taking heterosexual *a priori* as a starting point. However, the difficult position in which Lacan finds himself when he evokes a certain "ambiguity" in the Oedipus complex, reread in terms of the phallic signifier, can still perhaps be seen as one such *a priori*. In fact, during his famous address in Rome, in 1953, which gave a step-by-step account of the advances made by Freud, Lacan did not hesitate to tie the Oedipus complex to the influence of language in so far as it marks the "limits our discipline assigns to subjectivity."[64] Lacan turns this into a symbolic law: "This law, then, reveals itself clearly enough as identical to a language order."[65] This law is passed on, from generation to generation by the Name-of-the-Father. With the brilliance that is characteristic of his style, Lacan writes: "It is in the *name of the father* that we must recognize the basis of the symbolic function which, since the dawn of historical time, has identified his person with the figure of the law."[66] Even though everything plays out in the symbolic field, the terms employed are more than a little revealing.

On two occasions, and not without malice, Butler seizes upon the ambiguities and the complexities of Lacan's turn of phrase. She thus unpicks the certainty with which the Oedipal is tied to phallic signification. She cautions us against heteronormativity. Let us take a closer look at her approach.

Butler first tackles the subject of the Lacanian phallus in *Gender Trouble*. There, she criticizes Lacan's vision of the immutability of the symbolic order and the role which the phallus plays therein. We can very well put forth the real difference between the organ itself and the signifier of signifiers. We can very well assert the metaphoric dimension of Lacan's undertaking. We can furthermore underline the interest of reading Oedipus as a series of states that we can occupy and not as a concrete reality. Nevertheless: the choice of the terminology in and of itself, the semantic slippage which results, the connotations which flow forth from the vocabulary that is employed, all are worthy of investigation, dissection, and even a degree of ridicule, given that the place and the role of that which does not seem to be what it is appears to be decisive for the unconscious.

In fact, according to Butler, the symbolic must not be perceived as a monolithic block that accords us access to humanity. If "the symbolic order creates [...] intelligibility"[67] Lacan's question thus amounts to asking, "How is 'being' instituted and allocated through the signifying practices of the paternal economy?"[68] Butler's goal is quite clearly to renegotiate such a version of the symbolic, to lighten its framework, to illustrate its fallibility, to foreground its perpetual reconstruction through an analysis of social norms. "If the Symbolic is understood as a culturally universal structure of signification that is nowhere fully instantiated in the real, it makes sense to ask: What or who is it that signifies what or whom in this ostensibly crosscultural affair?"[69] In a subsequent book, Butler affirms, "Lacan remarks that the symbolic agencies crosscut differences among societies as the structure of an unconscious radically irreducible to social life."[70] In reality, according to Butler, one must leave space for the "flexibility of the Law itself, its cultural reformulation in more plastic forms [...]."[71] In particular if this has the pretention of determining the intelligibility of our very being. The invariable symbolic always runs the risk of erecting itself as an invariable instance which "promote[s] cultural stasis as its result."[72]

Like it or not, it is evident that by reading Lacan's text, *The Signification of the Phallus*, [73] word for word, we see the dialectic of the phallus of having (on the masculine side) and of being (on the feminine side), establishing the symbolic dimension of our existence through an orientation that is not only binary (possession or absence) but also resolutely heterosexual. This matters to Butler in so far as, for her, it affirms the fact that the totality of Lacan's work in reappropriating Freud does nothing more than ratify the "law of heterosexual desire."[74] Such a law exercises a violent injustice upon minority groups: it sidelines those who wish to couple by other means than through the possibilities that are available within the heterosexual norms. If the functioning of the unconscious can be explained in terms of a binary and heterosexual polarisation, how can it illuminate, without always already disqualifying homosexuals, trans, and the ambiguous who flourish outside of the *straight* and narrow?

At every step in her line of reasoning, Butler thus decides to undermine Lacan's thought process. Her interpretation highlights the comedic aspects of his model. "Both positions of 'having' and 'being' are, in Lacan's terms, finally to be understood as comedic failures that are nevertheless compelled to articulate and enact these repeated impossibilities."[75] In short, if we believe too strongly in the symbolic, if we raise it to the level of an ontology, if we take it as the sole transcultural guarantor, if we transform it into the only bulwark of desire (where the desire of the man who *has* the phallus is always strictly aroused by the woman who *is* the phallus), our sense of humour fails us. We blind ourselves in the light of the comedy of the sexes. We believe too strongly in one, and only one, formula through which the subject and its desire come about. We forget the offset undertaken by poststructuralism.[76] Butler cannot and does not want to let this legacy slide. Her theoretic work, as a whole, is undertaken "with the consequence that all gender ontology is reducible to the play of appearances."[77] She thus amuses herself in joyfully dragging Lacan far from the oppressiveness of being, the weight of the irrevocable, and in the direction of masquerade and pretence.

Butler's words echo deeply for those who envisage the psychoanalytic clinic from an exclusively Oedipal point of view where the latter, taken together with the Name-of-the-Father, form the foundation of the order of civilization.[78] Her philosophy develops a veritable devalorisation of the symbolic. The exclusive use of the Law of language, its "claim to be cultural intelligibility in its present and hegemonic form" is "ideologically suspect."[79] Body and language do not only encounter each other in our personal lives but are more generally inscribed within the cultural matrix that renders one or another form of life a life worth living, desirable or, on the contrary, pathological, inacceptable, and morally reprehensible.

On more than one occasion, Butler lingers on the fact that the positions designated by the phallus within the signifying chain are untenable and impossible. She thus concludes: "The construction of the law that guarantees failure is symptomatic of a slave morality that disavows the very generative powers it uses to construct the 'Law' as a permanent impossibility."[80] The heterosexual comedy, as ruled by the symbolic, results in a "slave morality." At bottom, following Foucault, Butler asks psychoanalysis – once the latter has had the clairvoyance to perceive the advent of humanity through the signifier – to unceasingly re-enact the conditions through which this humanity was established. In other words, she calls for us to turn away from this "slave morality," subject to the univocity of one and only one Law, and to turn toward what we could call an *ethics of the liberated body*, that is to say, an openness to the pluralisation of what is possible, liveable, desirable, beginning with the diversity of bodies and the diversity of ties that bind our bodies to language. While it is necessary for the ordering of the world, the edict of the symbolic Law must, nevertheless, take the bodies that it marks into account. Without this constant symbolic renegotiation, the establishment of such a Law risks not only the castration of the penis, but also, in their entirety, that of the bodies of those who are not able to introduce themselves into the self-evidence and the normality of a society based on the phallic opposition between "those who have it" and "those who lack it."

Butler's second reading of Lacan

In *Bodies That Matter, On the Discursive Limits of "Sex"* Butler takes up, for a second time, the question of the phallus in the Lacanian text. Once again, she is interested in phallic failure: the impossibility of characterizing the question of intelligibility and access to language through the phallic dialectic. What troubles Butler, and quite a few feminists, is that the "male genitals are suddenly themselves an originary site of erotogenization which then subsequently becomes the occasion for a set of substitutions or displacements."[81] The least evident substitution is that of the distinction between the penis and the phallus. Can we escape from the semantic shift that goes from one to the other? Moreover, making the phallus the originating symbol of the mark that language leaves upon our bodies in the context of a symbolic triangularization of desire proves to be problematic in so far as the starting point, the unsaid preconception of this elevation to an interplay of functions and sites remains, for once and for all, the strictly heterosexual couple. Seen from this angle, the symbolic dimension, just like that of the Oedipal, the phallus just like desire which it spurs on, the subject just like their access to the unconscious, all become mere tools that are used to tackle the drives from a *straight* point of view. Butler voluntarily tortures the Lacanian text. What of gender if, in place of Oedipus, we take hold of Antigone as the heroine of desire? What of a law "with no generality and no transposability?"[82] What of the symbolic if, in place of the phallus, and in following Luce Irigaray, we were to interest ourselves in the "'mechanics' of fluids,"[83] that is to say in a resolutely feminine writing? What of the political consequences on the family if the incest taboo had only been taken into account in order to exclude forms of parenthood alternative to that of the heterosexual couple? What of the phallus if our starting point, for the explanation of access to language, is not a heterosexually centred representation, but rather that of a lesbian couple?

Once again, there is no lack of derision. Once again, Butler laments and picks apart, in a particularly feminist manner, the ties that tacitly bind phallic signification to biological mimesis. Why does symbolic valency, the invention of an intelligible matrix independent from the reality of the sexes and of nature, still have to go through, not only the Oedipal, but also through the phallic as barometer?

From a clinical point of view, interrogating the question of the phallic in these terms is tantamount to interrogating the distinction between neuroses/psychoses in so far as the relation to the phallus and the path through the Oedipal constitute the primary reference point of diagnostic distinction. As Butler explains in an interview published in the journal *Radical Philosophy*: "I wanted to suggest that having and being are not mutually exclusive positions, and that there are a variety of identificatory possibilities that get animated within homosexuality and heterosexuality and bisexuality, which cannot easily be reduced to that particular framework."[84] We have, from her point of view, seen an idealization of masculine anatomy by means of the phallus.

> It seems that this imaginary valorization of body parts is to be derived from a kind of eroticized hypochondria. Hypochondria is an imaginary investment which [...] constitutes a libidinal projection of the body-surface which in turn establishes its epistemological accessibility.

> Hypochondria here denotes something like a *theatrical* delineation or production of the body, one which gives imaginary contours to the ego itself, projecting a body which becomes the occasion of an identification which in its imaginary or projected status is fully tenuous.[85]

The figure of the lesbian phallus undermines the masculine operation of the relationship to language. It does not deny the importance of the shift to the symbolic but demonstrates to what degree this insistence, as necessary, is not any less fundamentally fragile.

Variations on continual encryption

The trace that language leaves upon the body represents a decisive point when taken into account as a site of suffering and of expression. But such a site can always be re-signified. It is a site of multiple, or even plural plays. The theatre of the body is not only that of Artaud's body without organs, nor is it limited to the idealized recital of the Oedipal tragedy under the aegis of the phallus.

The possibility of experiencing one's body does not solely depend on one's organs. The vocabulary through which the body is described orientates its edification. Thus, when we take a new look at the words which describe the operational logic, the perception of the body is transformed. We could hazard a guess that the same is also true for the unconscious. In psychoanalysis, as in queer theory, the body can be considered as the site of inscription within language. For Lacan, reading Freud word for word, "It is the world of words that creates the world of things."[86] The materiality of the body is thus not only composed of skin and bones, of blood and fluids, but also of significations. For Butler, such significations cannot be exclusively determined by access to language through the phallus and the resolution of the Oedipal question.

The tension between words and things, between language and body, the ties between speech and sexuality, exceed the semantic slippage which leads from penis to phallus. The work of Butler's re-reading leads to "variable modes of delineating and theatricalizing body surfaces."[87] Bodies encode themselves when twisted by language, but Butler's reading results in a continuous variation of this encryption.

Her reading thus attenuates the violence which is characteristic of (hetero) normative exclusion, where the latter enjoys an unconscious epistemological advantage from the moment that the signification of the body is limited to the signification of the phallus. Here all genitives express a simultaneous double valency. Butler writes, "What is excluded from the body for the body's boundary to form?"[88] If it is clear that in terms of Lacanian signification, the phallus as the signifier of signifiers is always excluded from itself, to what degree does this self-exclusion, once it has asserted itself as all powerful within the symbolic regime, not eclipse others? Reflecting upon the signification of the phallus does not signify reflecting upon the meaning of the phallus, but rather on how meaning is brought forth from the phallus. Yet is it necessary that meaning stems from the idealization of this particular organ alone? Why not from others?

Butler's reading of Lacan is therefore salutary on at least two accounts: one, she pushes the thorny boundaries of the Freudian Lacanian logic, and two, her critiques allow for other significations of the body to be envisaged. These new significations are, of course, not exclusively phallic: they go far beyond slave morality. "It is unclear to me that lesbians can be said to be 'of' the same sex or that homosexuality in general ought to be construed as love of the same. If sex is always schematized in this sense, then there is no necessary reason for it to remain the same for all women."[89]

Beyond simply calling anatomy into question, what is sketched out here is the possibility to resignify the body, gender, sexuality, and meaning itself, independent from the phallic as the sole guiding light. Such an opening up of meaning includes an ironic reconsideration, an internal trituration and grinding up of the psychoanalytic discourse. In remaining unwary, in accepting too quickly, the impetus of metonymic slippages and the metaphorical jumps ends up excluding sexual minorities. Butler's irony requires that psychoanalytic discourse finds the words capable of decentring a number of its theoretic foundations. In thus tearing apart the underlying metapsychology, she pushes it to reinvent itself from the point of view of what it has hitherto considered as marginal.

In her two essays regarding the phallus, Butler closes with the question of the construction of gender and, twice, she maintains the location of the "process of gender incorporation within the wider orbit of melancholy."[90] The hypothesis of the melancholy of gender is as fundamental as it is complex in Butler's thought and has often been eclipsed by another thesis by which gender could be performative. I will return to both of these aspects.[91] For the moment, let us keep in mind that if we follow the Freudian Lacanian logic to the letter, the construction of gender, both masculine and feminine, necessitates the incest taboo. The melancholy of gender develops an idea according to which, before even being able to institute this taboo, the Freudian Lacanian logic is required to erect another: that against homosexuality.

In fact, when Butler characterizes the acquisition of gender in terms of melancholy, she undertakes a particularly *queer* reversal. In associating the construction of normal, adult, stable, completed sexual identity as stemming forth from melancholy, that is the "process of internalizing [...] lost loves,"[92] she succeeds in completely evacuating homophobia from the analytic discourse. She inverts the heteronormative matrix that she condemns. This is what we shall see in the following chapters. Beyond Oedipus, heteronormativity is excised from metapsychology which can thus reach out and challenge the invariance of *the* difference between the sexes.

Among the ruins of Oedipus

To work on the post-Oedipal scene, between queer theory and psychoanalysis is to thus undertake a double movement. On the one hand, this amounts to asking oneself to what degree heteronormativity and male dominance remain at work in our occidental societies and in our unconscious. One might as well state, and reiterate, that together with queer theory, psychoanalysis advances in the direction of a post-Oedipal scene if, and only if, its investigations of the drives are no longer grounded in heterosexual presumptions. What is at stake is not only ethical and epistemological but also institutional. The study of the human psyche must set aside any and all references to a norm that may in turn correspond to an ideal promising fulfilment, accomplishment, or happiness. It amounts, on the contrary, to making do with the characteristic disfunction of the *parlêtre*, "speech is a form of cancer that afflicts the human being." For Lacan, "speech is a parasite."[93]

On the other hand, it remains to be emphasized that, even in a post-Oedipal era, psychoanalysis still plays the grand theatre of gender against the real. The costumes and the games, the masks and the semblances, the rejoinders and silences, the slogans and gestures, the tragic just like the comic, the play just like the performance, all exist for a mere instant, so as to trick the void that spurs us on.

Beginning with Freud, psychoanalysis has perceived humanity as being grounded in a sombre excess. This hypothesis, even if relatively disheartening, has not lost its edge. Each subject, no matter the advances in society, no matter the avenues that have been opened up or the progress that has been made, has to confront, within the psyche itself, the repetition of something that refuses any satisfaction and all positivity. The drive denies the ideality of beauty, goodness, and truth. It insists. There are no better days to come, nor identitarian certitudes when faced with the repetition of the same.[94]

Faced with that which is impossible to endure, the analytic act alleviates through a strange paradox. Interpretation as an act, even though it requires a particular enunciative context, together with strictly established roles, is able to reconfigure the enunciative regime. The consequences of the interpretative act, when carefully aimed, allow the subject to hear what he has said, enabling him to take alternative actions. Post-Oedipal analysts whine when faced with the transformations of contemporary life. Their ambition does not include the systematic destruction of every scene and a militant return to the anoedipal factory. Rather, they impose upon themselves the task of uncovering the manner in which representation functions for the subjects to whom they lend their ears. What type of performance are they dealing with? In what genealogy are their gestures, bodies, and voices inscribed? And, most important of all, how do they stage their existence? To each his role in the great theatre of gender. Locating the workings of the drive thus means situating where the gap, the blank, and that which dismantles the memory of text and liberates desire, appear.

Upon the ruins of Oedipus and of the phallus, an awareness, a practice and an ethics continue to be invented, in the light of the real. We must now clarify somewhat the manner in which this awareness, this practice and these ethics are laid out, and how they manage to avoid the pitfalls of homophobia and heteronormativity. It also remains to be seen whether (or not) such an ethics, such a practice and such an awareness lead us beyond *the* difference between the sexes.

Notes

1 During the debates concerning "le mariage pour tous" ("marriage for all," the legalization of same sex marriage in France in 2013), a petition by "Psychoanalysts regarding equal rights and 'le Mariage pour Tous'" ("Des psychanalystes face à l'égalité des droits au 'Mariage pour tous'") stated that it is not the role of psychoanalysis to be moralizing and prescriptive ("[il] ne revient pas à la psychanalyse de se montrer moralisatrice et prédictive"). Jacques-Alain Miller, in turn, circulated a petition which argued against the instrumentalization of psychoanalysis, remarking that the Oedipal structure uncovered by Freud is not invariant in anthropological terms ("la structure oedipienne dégagée par Freud n'est pas un invariant anthropologique"). To other ends, Eric Fassin sketches out a detailed map of the unfortunate public statements made by certain analyts, see Eric Fassin, *L'Inversion de la question homosexuelle* (Editions Amsterdam, 2008). See also the essay by Thamy Ayouch, "Psychanalyse et mauvais genre: la tentation de l'ontologie," in *Masqereading: comment faire des études-genres avec la literature*, ed. Guyonne Leduc (L'Harmattan, 2014), 89–102.

2 Sigmund Freud, "Extracts from the Fliess Papers: Letter 71 (October 15, 1897)" in *The Standard Edition of the Complete Psychological Works of Sigmund Freud*. Vol. I. Edited by James Strachey, Anna Freud, and Angela Richards. (Hogarth Press, 1953–1974), 265.

3 Herman Nunberg, *Principles of Psychoanalysis: Their Application to the Neuroses*, trans. Madlyn Kahr and Sidney Kahr (International Universities Press, 1955), 70.

4 Sigmund Freud, "The Question of Lay Analysis" in *The Standard Edition of the Complete Psychological Works of Sigmund Freud*. Vol. XX, 212. Freud, more precisely, refers in English in his text, to the monograph by the explorer Henry Morgan Stanley, *Through the Dark Continent*, published in 1879.

5 Herman Nunberg, *Principles of Psychoanalysis: Their Application to the Neuroses*, 68.

6 Among other texts, see Monique Plaza, "'Phallomorphic' power and the psychology of 'woman,'" *Feminist Issues*, 1, (1980): 71–102, doi: 10.1007/BF02685560. For perspectives on feminist critiques of psychoanalysis before the advent of queer theory see Juliet Mitchell, *Psychoanalysis and Feminism* (Vintage Books, 1975).

7 For Aristotle, Sophocles' Oedipus Rex constitutes an unsurpassed model of coherent and credible narration, see Aristotle, "Poetics," in *The Complete Works of Aristotle*, Vol. II, ed. Jonathan Barnes (Princeton University Press, 1984), 1452a (2323) and 1454a (2326). Paul Ricoeur drew on the consequences of Aristotle's *Poetics* in Paul Ricoeur, *Time and Narrative*, Vol. I, trans. Kathleen McLauglin and David Pellauer (University of Chicago Press, 1983). The consequences for

psychoanalysis are discussed in Paul Ricoeur, *On Psychoanalysis, Writings and Lectures*, Vol. I, trans. David Pellauer (Polity Press, 2012).

8 In the light of the image that Lacan uses in "The highway and the signifier 'being a father.'" See Jacques Lacan, *The Psychoses. The Seminar of Jacques Lacan. Book III 1955–1956*, ed. Jacques-Alain Miller, trans. Russell Grigg (Routledge, 1993), 285–195.

9 Let us remember that in Monique Wittig, *Le Corps lesbien* (Minuit, 1973) all of the mute *e* of the French personal pronouns were highlighted through the use of "/e" as a writing convention. This rendered the text not only far less intelligible but starkly drew attention to the insufferable silence of the feminine within the context of the alleged neutrality of contemporary, and entirely phallogocentric, language. See also, Monique Wittig, *The Lesbian Body*, trans. David Le Vay (Beacon Press, 1986).

10 Monique Wittig, "The Straight Mind" in *The Straight Mind and Other Essays* (Beacon Press, 1992), 22.

11 Gilles Deleuze has written a particularly valuable essay which illustrates the functioning of the symbolic order, see Gilles Deleuze, "How Do We Recognize Structuralism?" in *Desert Islands and Other Texts 1953–1974*, ed. David Lapoujade, trans. Michael Taormina (Semiotext(e), 2004), 170–189.

12 Monique Wittig, "The Straight Mind," 28.

13 Monique Wittig, "The Category of Sex" in *The Straight Mind and Other Essays* (Beacon Press, 1992), 4.

14 Monique Wittig, "The Straight Mind," 25.

15 See Jacques Lacan, "The Signification of the Phallus" in *Écrits*, trans. Bruce Fink (W.W. Norton & Company, 2006), 575–584.

16 Monique Wittig, "The Straight Mind," 27–28.

17 See Monique Wittig, *Le corps lesbian.*

18 See Monique Wittig and Sande Zeig, *Lesbian Peoples, Material for a Dictionary* (Avon Books, 1979).

19 For example, the anthropologist Françoise Héritier does not hesitate to qualify it as "the ultimate buffer of thought." For her "the observation of the difference between the sexes is the foundation of all thought, traditional as well as scientific." See Françoise Héritier, "Masculine/Feminine: The Thought of Difference," in *Contemporary French Feminism*, ed. Kelly Olivier and Lisa Walsh (Oxford University Press, 2004), 59.

20 See the work of Didier Éribon, *Hérésies. Essais sur a théorie de la sexualité* (Fayard, 2003). See also Didier Éribon, *Insult and the Making of the Gay Self*, trans. Michael Lucey (Duke University Press, 2004).

21 Monique Wittig, "The Straight Mind," 32.

22 Monique Wittig and Sande Zeig, *Lesbian Peoples, Material for a Dictionary*, 157.

23 Monique Wittig, "Paradigm," in *Homosexualities and French Literature: Cultural Contexts, Critical Texts*, ed. George Stambolian and Elaine Marks, trans. George Stambolian (Cornell University Press, 1979), 119.

24 "[The question] is rather a matter of challenging the pervasive culture of psychology in modernity, the popular practices and discourses of psychology (that is, psychology with a small *p*), along with their disciplinary, academic base in depth psychology, personality psychology, the psychological sciences of the individual. The goal is not to discredit psychology as an intellectual project so much as to escape a style of thinking that understands the person in terms of individual interiority and judges subjective life according to a normative standard of healthy functioning." David Halperin, *What Do Gay Men Want? An Essay on Sex, Risk and Subjectivity* (University of Michigan Press, 2007), 9. I will return, in the

following chapter, and in more detail to David Halperin's insights in order to undo homophobia within the psyche. Let us for the time being content ourselves in remarking, on one hand, the proximity of his project to that of the anti-Oedipal critics, even if his principle point of reference is Foucault, and, on the other hand, the synonymy which appears later in his essay concerning psychology, the self, and psychoanalysis. Such equivalences are, to my mind, not quite so self-evident.

25 Gilles Deleuze and Félix Guattari, *Kafka, Towards a Minor Literature*, trans. Dana Polan (University of Minnesota Press, 1986), 82.

26 Gilles Deleuze and Félix Guattari, *Anti-Oedipus Capitalism and Schizophrenia*, trans. Robert Hurley, Mark Seem and Helen R. Lane (University of Minnesota Press, 1983), 314.

27 Gilles Deleuze and Félix Guattari, *Anti-Oedipus Capitalism and Schizophrenia*, 23.

28 Sigmund Freud, "The Interpretation of Dreams" in *The Standard Edition of the Complete Psychological Works of Sigmund Freud*. Vol. IV, 536.

29 Sigmund Freud, "The Interpretation of Dreams," 48.

30 Sigmund Freud, "The Interpretation of Dreams," 261.

31 Sigmund Freud, "The Interpretation of Dreams," 261.

32 Sigmund Freud, "The Interpretation of Dreams," 261.

33 Gilles Deleuze and Félix Guattari, *Anti-Oedipus Capitalism and Schizophrenia*, 311.

34 Gilles Deleuze and Félix Guattari, *Anti-Oedipus Capitalism and Schizophrenia*, 380.

35 Gilles Deleuze and Félix Guattari, *Anti-Oedipus Capitalism and Schizophrenia*, 9.

36 Gilles Deleuze and Félix Guattari, *Anti-Oedipus Capitalism and Schizophrenia*, 46.

37 The references to this point in the work of Deleuze and Guattari are far too numerous to count. One could however consider a point of departure as being: Gilles Deleuze and Félix Guattari, *A Thousand Plateaus. Capitalism and Schizophrenia*, trans. Brian Massumi (University of Minnesota Press, 1987), 208–232.

38 Gilles Deleuze and Félix Guattari, *Anti-Oedipus Capitalism and Schizophrenia*, 310.

39 Gilles Deleuze and Félix Guattari, *Anti-Oedipus Capitalism and Schizophrenia*, 83–84.

40 Gilles Deleuze, *Essays Critical and Clinical*, trans. Daniel W. Smith and Michael A. Greco (University of Minnesota Press, 1997), 4.

41 Gilles Deleuze and Félix Guattari, *Anti-Oedipus Capitalism and Schizophrenia*, 274.

42 "Where Id was, there Ego shall be." Sigmund Freud, "New Introductory Lectures on Psychoanalysis" in *The Standard Edition of the Complete Psychological Works of Sigmund Freud*. Vol. XXII, 80.

43 This is what Lacan perfectly understands when he translates Oedipus as the "Name-of-the-Father," in French "le nom-du-père," which plays on the homonymy of "nom" or "name" and "non" or "no." See Jacques Lacan, *Formations of the Unconscious. The Seminar of Jacques Lacan. Book V 1957–1958*, ed. Jacques-Alain Miller, trans. Russell Grigg (Polity, 2017), 163–197.

44 Gayle Rubin "The Traffic in Women: Notes on the Political Economy of Sex" in *Toward an Anthropology of Women*, ed. Rayna R. Reiter, (Monthly Review Press, 1975), 189.

45 Gilles Deleuze and Félix Guattari, *Anti-Oedipus Capitalism and Schizophrenia*, 366. All of Deleuze and Guattari's work tends, for that matter, to agree with the immanent plenitude of life that encompasses all that is experienced so as to open each individuality to the impersonal and the multiple. As one of his final texts

illustrates: "a life should not have to be enclosed in the simple moment when individual life confronts universal death. *A life* is everywhere, in every moment which a living subject traverses." And further on in the same text: "'A' or 'An' (one) is always the index of a multiplicity: an event, a singularity, a life…" See, Gilles Deleuze, *Two Regimes of Madness. Texts and Interviews 1975–1995*, ed. David Lapoujade, trans. Ames Hodges and Mike Taormina (Semiotext(e), 2006), 387–388.

46 Gilles Deleuze and Félix Guattari, *Anti-Oedipus Capitalism and Schizophrenia*, 293.

47 Gilles Deleuze and Félix Guattari, *Anti-Oedipus Capitalism and Schizophrenia*, 294.

48 Gilles Deleuze and Félix Guattari, *Anti-Oedipus Capitalism and Schizophrenia*, 293.

49 Gilles Deleuze and Félix Guattari, *Anti-Oedipus Capitalism and Schizophrenia*, 295.

50 Gilles Deleuze and Félix Guattari, *Anti-Oedipus Capitalism and Schizophrenia*, 271.

51 This approach is at the heart of the final chapter.

52 This is the subject of the excellent contribution of Manola Antonioli. See Manola Antonioli, "Mapping the Unconscious" in *Why Guattari? A Liberation of Cartographies, Ecologies and Politics*, ed. Thomas Jellis, Joe Gerlach, and John-David Dewsbury (Routledge, 2019), 34–45.

53 "nel regime del Nome-del-Padre egli esce dall'indeterminazione e viene inscritto sotto una significazione precisa, la significazione fallica, che è il prodotto del significante paterno sul bambino." Antonio Di Ciaccia and Massimo Recalcati, *Jacques Lacan: un insegnamento sul sapere dell'inconscio* (Mondadori, 2000), 98.

54 Jacques Lacan, *Formations of the Unconscious*, 223.

55 Jacques Lacan, "The Signification of the Phallus," in *Écrits*, trans. Bruce Fink (W. W. Norton & Company, 2006), 581.

56 Jacques Lacan, *Formations of the Unconscious*, 267.

57 Jacques Lacan, *Formations of the Unconscious*, 146.

58 Jacques Lacan, *Formations of the Unconscious*, 319.

59 Jacques Lacan, *Formations of the Unconscious*, 149.

60 Judith Butler, *Gender Trouble: Feminism and the Subversion of Identity* (Routledge, 1999), 22.

61 Judith Butler, "An interview with Judith Butler," *The Believer*, May 1, 2003, https://www.thebeliever.net/an-interview-with-judith-butler/

62 Judith Butler, *Gender Trouble: Feminism and the Subversion of Identity* (Routledge, 1999), viii.

63 Judith Butler, "An interview with Judith Butler."

64 Jacques Lacan, "The Function and Field of Speech and Language in Psychoanalysis," in *Écrits*, 229.

65 Jacques Lacan, "The Function and Field of Speech and Language in Psychoanalysis," in *Écrits*, 229.

66 Jacques Lacan, "The Function and Field of Speech and Language in Psychoanalysis," in *Écrits*, 230.

67 Judith Butler, *Gender Trouble*, 56.

68 Judith Butler, *Gender Trouble*, 56.

69 Judith Butler, *Gender Trouble*, 57.

70 Judith Butler, *Antigone's Claim. Kinship Between Life and Death* (Columbia University Press, 2000), 44.

71 Judith Butler, *Gender Trouble*, 72.

72 Judith Butler, *Gender Trouble*, 71.
73 Jacques Lacan, "The Signification of the Phallus," in *Écrits*, 575–585.
74 Judith Butler, *Gender Trouble*, 80.
75 Judith Butler, *Gender Trouble*, 59.
76 Judith Butler, *Gender Trouble*, 57.
77 Judith Butler, *Gender Trouble*, 60.
78 See, for instance, the numerous statements by Jean-Pierre Winter, in Jean-Pierre Winter, *Homoparenté. Naître de parents de même sexe* (Albin Michel, 2010).
79 Judith Butler, *Gender Trouble*, 72.
80 Judith Butler, *Gender Trouble*, 73.
81 Judith Butler, *Bodies That Matter, On the Discursive Limits of "Sex"* (Routledge, 1993), 60.
82 Judith Butler, *Antigone's Claim*, 10.
83 See Luce Irigaray, "The 'Mechanics' of Fluids" in *This Sex Which is not One*, trans. Catherine Porter and Carolyn Burke (Cornell University Press, 1985), 106–118.
84 Judith Butler, "Gender as Performance: An Interview with Judith Butler," *Radical Philosophy* 67 (Summer 1994), 37.
85 Judith Butler, *Bodies That Matter*, 63.
86 Jacques Lacan, "The Function and Field of Speech and Language in Psychoanalysis," in *Écrits*, 229.
87 Judith Butler, *Bodies That Matter*, 64.
88 Judith Butler, *Bodies That Matter*, 65.
89 Judith Butler, *Bodies That Matter*, 65–66.
90 Judith Butler, *Gender Trouble*, 64.
91 I will be considering the performative in the following chapter which the question of the melancholy of gender is considered in chapter IV.
92 Judith Butler, *Gender Trouble*, 74.
93 Jacques Lacan, *The Sinthome. The Seminar of Jacques Lacan. Book XXIII 1975–1976*, ed. Jacques-Alain Miller, trans. A.R. Price (Polity, 2016), 78
94 Regarding the negative dimension of the subject as approached by psychoanalysis, see Jacques Lacan, "Science and Truth" in *Écrits*, 726–745. See also Lee Edelman, *No Future, Queer Theory and the Death Drive* (Duke University Press, 2004), notably Chapter 1, "The Future is Kid Stuff."

Bibliography

Antonioli, Manola. "Mapping the Unconscious." In: *Why Guattari? A Liberation of Cartographies, Ecologies and Politics.* Edited by Thomas Jellis, Joe Gerlach and John-David Dewsbury. Routledge, 2019, 27–36.

Aristotle, "Poetics," in *The Complete Works of Aristotle.* Vol. II. Edited by Jonathan Barnes. Princeton University Press, 1984.

Ayouch, Thamy. "Psychanalyse et mauvais genre: la tentation de l'ontologie." In: *Masqereading: comment faire des études-genres avec la literature*, edited by Guyonne Leduc. L'Harmattan, 2014, 89–102.

Butler, Judith. *Bodies That Matter, On the Discursive Limits of "Sex."*Routledge, 1993.

Butler, Judith. "Gender as Performance: An Interview with Judith Butler," *Radical Philosophy* 67 (Summer 1994): 32–39.

Butler, Judith. *Gender Trouble: Feminism and the Subversion of Identity*. Routledge, 1999.
Butler, Judith. *Antigone's Claim. Kinship Between Life and Death*. Columbia University Press, 2000.
Butler, Judith. "An Interview with Judith Butler," *The Believer*. May 1, 2003. https://www.thebeliever.net/an-interview-with-judith-butler/.
Deleuze, Gilles. *Essays Critical and Clinical*. Translated by Daniel W. Smith and Michael A. Greco. University of Minnesota Press, 1997.
Deleuze, Gilles. "How Do We Recognize Structuralism?" in *Desert Islands and Other Texts 1953–1974*. Edited by David Lapoujade. Translated by Michael Taormina. Semiotext(e), 2004, 170–189.
Deleuze, Gilles. *Two Regimes of Madness. Texts and Interviews 1975–1995*. Edited by David Lapoujade. Translated by Ames Hodges and Michael Taormina. Semiotext (e), 2006, 387–388.
Deleuze, Gilles and Félix Guattari. *Anti-Oedipus Capitalism and Schizophrenia*. Translated by Robert Hurley, Mark Seem and Helen R. Lane. University of Minnesota Press, 1983, 314.
Deleuze, Gilles and Félix Guattari. *Kafka, Towards a Minor Literature*. Translated by Dana Polan. University of Minnesota Press, 1986.
Deleuze, Gilles and Félix Guattari, *A Thousand Plateaus. Capitalism and Schizophrenia*. Translated by Brian Massumi. University of Minnesota Press, 1987.
Di Ciaccia, Antonio and Massimo Recalcati, *Jacques Lacan: un insegnamento sul sapere dell'inconscio*. Mondadori, 2000.
Edelman, Lee. *No Future, Queer Theory and the Death Drive*. Duke University Press, 2004.
Éribon, Didier. *Hérésies. Essais sur a théorie de la sexualité*. Fayard, 2003.
Éribon, Didier. *Insult and the Making of the Gay Self*. Translated by Michael Lucey. Duke University Press, 2004.
Fassin, Eric. *L'Inversion de la question homosexuelle*. Editions Amsterdam, 2008.
Freud, Sigmund. *The Standard Edition of the Complete Psychological Works of Sigmund Freud*. Edited by James Strachey, Anna Freud, and Angela Richards. Hogarth Press, 1953–1974.
Halperin, David. *What Do Gay Men Want? An Essay on Sex, Risk and Subjectivity*. University of Michigan Press, 2007.
Héritier, Françoise. "Masculine/Feminine: The Thought of Difference." In *Contemporary French Feminism*. Edited by Kelly Olivier and Lisa Walsh. Oxford University Press, 2004, 56–73.
Irigaray, Luce. "The 'Mechanics' of Fluids." In *This Sex Which is Not One*. Translated by Catherine Porter and Carolyn Burke. Cornell University Press, 1985, 106–118.
Lacan, Jacques. *The Psychoses. The Seminar of Jacques Lacan. Book III 1955–1956*. Edited by Jacques-Alain Miller. Translated by Russell Grigg. Routledge, 1993.
Lacan, Jacques. *Écrits*. Translated by Bruce Fink. W.W. Norton & Company, 2006.
Lacan, Jacques. *The Sinthome. The Seminar of Jacques Lacan. Book XXIII 1975–1976* Edited by Jacques-Alain Miller. Translated by A.R. Price. Polity, 2016.
Lacan, Jacques. *Formations of the Unconscious. The Seminar of Jacques Lacan. Book V 1957–1958*. Edited by Jacques-Alain Miller. Translated by Russell Grigg. Polity, 2017.

Mitchell, Juliet. *Psychoanalysis and Feminism*. Vintage Books, 1975.
Nunberg, Herman. *Principles of Psychoanalysis: Their Application to the Neuroses.* Translated by: Madlyn Kahr and Sidney Kahr. International Universities Press, 1955.
Plaza, Monique. "'Phallomorphic' Power and the Psychology of 'Woman'," *Feminist Issues* 1 (1980): 71–102. doi:10.1007/BF02685560.
Ricoeur, Paul. *Time and Narrative.* Vol. I. Translated by Kathleen McLauglin and David Pellauer. University of Chicago Press, 1983.
Ricoeur, Paul. *On Psychoanalysis, Writings and Lectures.* Vol. I. Translated by David Pellauer. Polity Press, 2012.
Rubin, Gayle. "The Traffic in Women: Notes on the Political Economy of Sex." In *Toward an Anthropology of Women*. Edited by Rayna R. Reiter. Monthly Review Press, 1975.
Winter, Jean-Pierre. *Homoparenté. Naître de parents de même sexe.* Albin Michel, 2010.
Wittig, Monique. *Le corps lesbian*. Minuit, 1973.
Wittig, Monique. "Paradigm," in *Homosexualities and French Literature: Cultural Contexts, Critical Texts.* Edited by George Stambolian and Elaine Marks. Translated by George Stambolian. Cornell University Press, 1979, 114–121.
Wittig, Monique. *The Lesbian Body.* Translated by David Le Vay. Beacon Press, 1986.
Wittig, Monique. *The Straight Mind and Other Essays.* Beacon Press, 1992.
Wittig, Monique and Sande Zeig. *Lesbian Peoples, Material for a Dictionary.* Avon Books, 1979.

Chapter 3

Performing Homo-analysis

Fabrice Bourlez

A disturbing silence?

Ever since Freud penned his famous case, of the "young homosexual,"[1] a number of publications have testified to the interest that homosexuality holds for psychoanalysis. Even today, the clinic of homosexualities,[2] that of gays undergoing analysis,[3] the homosexual unconscious,[4] female homosexualities,[5] and homo-analysands,[6] constitute the many pieces of the foundation which, one after the other, continue to interrogate this fringe of sexual practice. At best, the need to take homosexuality into account in a post-Oedipal clinic capable of reinventing itself beyond any universalist reference becomes apparent, being nevertheless at the risk of once again succumbing to a stigmatizing conservatism that still associates homosexuality with perversion.[7] Indeed, a progressive destigmatization of homosexuality has seen the light of day within clinical literature. Yet, as regards practicians, will this movement, at once salutary and fruitful as concerns analysis, suffice in removing any suspicion of homophobia? Can we show that Freud and his metapsychology were *gay friendly*, as one says today?

When all is said and done, in all of these texts and publications, one question remains unresolved most of the time. It is, in fact, more than a question, it is a silence: something that the post-Oedipal clinic still has difficulty in formulating, that the clinic does not ask (itself), and that is only addressed on rare occasions. In short, a sort of latent "don't ask don't tell," to use the phrase most often associated with the American military and its practice of keeping the possible presence of homosexuals among the troops quiet.[8] Even the most enlightened post-Oedipal psychoanalysis does not often, or even at all, question itself as concerns the sexual orientation of the therapist.[9] As the practice of psychoanalysis has become more open and respectful on a case-by-case basis, more singularly focused on each individual subject, as the stigmatizing term of perversion has been used less and less often in order to (dis)qualify homosexuality, the question of homosexual psychoanalysts has likewise been the subject of less and less discussion. This silence may be synonymous with modernity or discretion. There is perhaps

DOI: 10.4324/9781003612735-3

little merit in this question in so far as it does not pose a problem to anyone, or perhaps because no one is interested in the answer. Perhaps.

Yet, in *Epistemology of the Closet*, Eve K. Sedgwick insists on the fact that remaining silent offers the other the right to not know, ignorance itself is always part of the stakes of a given power dynamic. The queer theorist thus inverses the hypothesis proposed by Michel Foucault according to which knowledge is never free and liberatory but inscribed within a power dynamic.[10] Not knowing is also power. It is therefore widely accepted, in occidental society, that we do not know how to speak an African dialect, that we do not know the name of the president of Peru, or, in on a different note, that we do not know whether such and such a cineast, or such and such a painter, member of the armed forces, or minister, is homosexual. On the contrary, it is difficult to be unaware of the (heterosexual) marriage of the Prince of Wales, or of the name of the President of the United States of America (and of that of his wife). According to Sedgwick, these blind spots, these dark zones of ignorance and secrecy, of unknowing, allow the dominant class to continue to exercise their prerogatives, and inversely, oblige others to continue to speak their languages, to be aware of their titles and their practices in the absence of any reciprocal interest.

Sedgwick's analysis, developed in the midst of the AIDS crisis sees itself as resolutely anti-homophobic. She constructs an epistemology, which, to say the least can be qualified as bizarre, by taking into account that curious and eternally reiterated speech act: coming out of the closet. What epistemological and political consequences can be ascribed to this unsaid, to this affirmation of preference, to this declaration of sexual orientation, to the dissolution of this stroke of ignorance? What happens when we put the other in a position in which it is impossible not to know? At that time, but it no doubt remains true today, the author remarked that

> The number of persons or institutions by whom the existence of gay people – never mind the existence of *more gay people* – is treated as a precious desideratum, a needed condition of life, is small, even compared to those who may wish for the dignified treatment of any gay people who happen to already exist.[11]

Here benevolent acceptation, affable tolerance, polite respect, no longer suffice. To rid society of its lingering homophobia is to recognize homosexuality not merely as something that is tolerable, admissible or conceivable, but as a desirable, valued way of life, a choice which is as normal as it is enviable.

The question can thus be stated in the following terms: does the analytic practice desire, or hope to see, not only gays and lesbians undergoing analysis, but gay and lesbian analysts? Turning the question of inversion on its head amounts to calling this unspoken aspect of the analytic milieu into question. What type of unknowing is hidden within? What power dynamics are anchored therein? Should we merely associate it with the well-meaning silence of the analyst's evenly suspended attention? Or does it lead elsewhere?

A decade after her singular and valuable statements regarding the civil solidarity pact (pacte civil de solidarité, PACS),[12] Sabine Prokhoris opened her work entitled *Insaisissable Histoire de la psychanalyse* [13] with a remark that is as disturbing as it is pertinent. She too acknowledges that the work of the analytic field concerning homosexualities, testifies, today, to a relative open-mindedness. It is clear that the equation linking homosexuality to perversion is not as immediate as it was at a certain time. But Prokhoris adds that this open-mindedness is not as clearly expressed when the subject of new modalities of filiation are raised. For example, what of the position of psychoanalysts concerning assisted reproductive technology and surrogacy? The call to an all-powerful symbolic order is quick to once again resound.

As Prokhoris explains,

> As for what concerns, in the practice of psychoanalytic associations beyond tolerance or good intentions, the admission of candidates for training, or member analysts who are homosexual and who can openly *say* so – transsexuals, supposing that the situation arises, let's not even get into that – cautious silence.[14]

In fact, other than in journal issues or in special editions dedicated to the question of homosexualities, this silence can be found throughout the various publications and theorizations dedicated to transference, countertransference, the subject supposed to know, the place that the analyst occupies within the cure as such, or the particular practice of the *pass.* [15] All of these elements nevertheless allow the *praxis* to lay claim to an "orientation." The lexical ambiguity of the latter term is, of course, of great interest here.

Reading these works, examining the space from which these reflexions are spoken, beginning with Freud's own original text which transformed his patient Sidonie Csillag into an eternally "young homosexual,"[16] the neutrality and the authority of those who offer their opinions on behalf of psychoanalysis is quite surprising. They are impartial, absolutist, detached from the stakes of minorities. To what degree does such authority and such neutrality depend upon an implicit position, grounded in strict heterosexuality and entirely polarized by the sacrosanct difference between the sexes?[17] Once more, and forgive my insistence on this point, understand that it is performative, what happens when "crazy" is confronted by "queer" in an analytic space? Would this non-thematization – a euphemism to be sure – be the synonym of an undeclared suspicion concerning the spectrum of homosexualities? In other words, and in echoing Monique Wittig, would *the orientation of the clinic* be fundamentally and constructively *straight* and, as a consequence, despite the best of intentions, somewhat homophobic? In not daring to ask this question in such explicit terms we allow uncertainty to persist.

But what if we were to reply in an irritated tone that the interest in the real, in the drives, the consideration of the above on a case-by-case basis shatters the distinction between homo and heterosexual so dear to Sedgwick? Is this type of challenge of any importance to the psychoanalytic clinic? Are we not mixing ourselves up in social issues in raising this type of non-issue? Have norms ever been of concern for the psyche? And why should the intimacy of the subject be disclosed differently depending on the sexual orientation of the analyst? For that matter, the analysands themselves, from their position on the analytic couch do not actually care at all about the sexual orientation of their analyst! What would such a revelation change? Where could such considerations take us? A simple solution lies upon the horizon "Stop asking just here; stop asking just now; we know in advance the kind of difference that could be made by the invocation of *this* difference; it makes no difference; it doesn't mean."[18] In point of fact, heterosexual analysts never declare their sexual preference in any of the clinical notes that they pen. On this matter, it is clear that no heterosexual has ever declared his heterosexuality. Let us remind ourselves that no heterosexual has *come out*: at no point, and under no circumstances has a heterosexual had to come out of the closet. It is neither necessary nor of any interest.[19] In short, pointing out this silence within the analytic milieu disturbs, seizes up the self-evident silence of the subject supposed to know, his humdrum caution as well as the discretion of his signifying attention.

For Sedgwick, "silence on these issues performs the enforcing work of the status quo more predictably and inexorably than any attempt at analysis."[20] To paint a clearer picture of what I mean, if the style of the analyst depends upon the tone of his enunciation, for the time being, the tones, even the most well-meaning, prove to be remarkably alike. They paint over all clinical testimonies with a *straight* varnish. This image is dominated by the presupposed heterosexuality of the clinicians, particularly when they treat cases of homosexuality, and let us not even get onto the topic of "transsexuality." In order to envisage leaving the status quo behind, post-Oedipal analysis needs to bring this revolution to fruition! If homo-analysands, trans-analysands, and queer-analysands, exist, do homo-analysts, trans-analysts, and queer-analysts? Instead of considering the discourse of the analysand, on the couch, in terms of expropriation, our difficulty can now be stated as follows: *is the analytic practice not a closet?*

This particular problematic imposes itself as voluntarily perverse, impertinent, inappropriate (but is the subject of desire necessarily conformist and polite?). It inscribes the observer in the tableau and raises the question of that which has hitherto remained unconsidered within the clinic, that is, an edge of the psychological field which perhaps deserves further investigation.

Sedgwick envisages coming out of the closet as a "performative space of contradiction."[21] Knowing or not knowing, coming out of the closet or staying in the closet, informs us not only as to the status of the person concerned by this linguistic trope, but also regarding the repercussions of these speech acts in general, what speaking means, and as concerns the capacity to do things with words.[22] In performative utterances, the epistemology of the closet finds a manner of disturbing the heterosexual suppositions at work in society: an utterance that, endlessly, should be repeated so as to destabilize the order, grammar, structures, and positions of enunciation. An approach which seeks to produce an outwardly utterance is worthy of praise as there are "few gay people, however courageous and forthright by habit, however fortunate is the support of their immediate communities, in whose lives the closet is not still a shaping presence."[23]

Moreover, in Sedgwick's writing we find the disappointment concerning psychoanalysis that we have already seen elsewhere:

> Psychoanalytic theory [...] seemed to promise to introduce a certain becoming amplitude into discussions of what different people are like – only to turn, in its streamlined trajectory across so many institutional boundaries, into the sveltest of metatheoretical disciplines, sleeked down to such elegant operational entities as *the* mother, *the* father, *the* pre-oedipal, *the* oedipal, *the other* or Other.[24]

Thus, and once more, psychoanalysis would have closed the door that led to the Outside.

Was Freud gay friendly?

A sneaking suspicion remains. It is difficult to clear away with a wave of one's hand. Is the clinician's psychoanalytic practice in league with whatever nondescript heteronormative power? Does analysis wring the ability of self-description and self-declaration away from homosexuality? And what if the neutrality of the psychoanalyst were little more than a mask that one is required to wear so as to embody the spectre of heterosexuality? If we were to respond in the affirmative to any of these questions the gap between analytic discourse and that of queer theory could not be more pronounced. The accusations of homophobia would be irrefutable.

In *Leonardo Da Vinci and a Memory of his Childhood* the two opposing points of view are clearly expressed.

> Homosexual men, who have in our times taken vigorous action against the restrictions imposed by law on their sexual activity, are fond of representing themselves, through their theoretical spokesmen, as being from the outset a distinct sexual species, as an intermediate sexual stage,

> as a "third sex." They are, they claim, men who are innately compelled by organic determinants to find pleasure in men and have been debarred from obtaining it in women. Much as one would be glad on grounds of humanity to endorse their claims, one must treat their theories with some reserve, for they have been advanced without regard for the physical genesis of homosexuality. *Psycho-analysis offers the means of filling this gap and of putting the assertions of homosexuals to the test.* It has succeeded in the task only in the case of a small number of persons, but all the investigations undertaken so far have yielded the same surprising result.[25]

This extract is as exasperating as it is gratifying. On one hand it is difficult to dispute Freud's attitude: he wants only the best for humanity, for each to be able to live the life that they would like. Freud is *friendly.* His theory seeks to appear as visionary, open, and subversive. We are, after all, in 1910.[26]

But on the other hand, it is equally difficult not to tense up when analytic understanding offhandedly repackages the theoretic advances, ideologies, and demands of homosexuals themselves. "Their theories [...] have been advanced without regard for the psychical genesis of homosexuality. Psycho-analysis offers the means of filling this gap and of putting the assertions of homosexuals to the test." In rereading this passage, one is struck by a singular question: by what right? Why would psychoanalysis know how to better express what is going on than those that are directly concerned? How could it better describe the state of affairs? To what degree can we detach the experience of stigmatization, of rejection, of fear, and of shame that certain homosexuals experience on a daily basis from the psychical genesis of homosexuality? Why does psychoanalysis need to fill the gap in the theories put forward by homosexuals? And why does it need to put these affirmations to the test? If psychoanalysis is to consider itself as always having the last word, if it is to position itself as that which states the truth of the matter, and if it were to call upon itself to fill the gaps, it risks saturating subjects with its knowledge, it risks adopting a view looking on from above,[27] overlooking the sidestep characteristic of its process and of its attentiveness.

In short, once again, the *gay friendly Freud*, expressed in a minor key, finds itself superposed against another, in a major key, authoritarian, transcendental, deaf to that which the homosexuals affirm. Do we really have any need for an explanation of this "sexual aberration," in terms employed in 1919, which did not offer sons "the correct decision in [their] choice of object, namely someone of the opposite sex?"[28] How, why, for whom, and with which criteria? Would these not be directly attributable to values or to morals? At bottom, when psychoanalysis raises the spectre of a "correct decision," does it not directly fall prey to the critique that it proposes as concerns theoreticians of homosexuality, that is: to work and pass judgement within the norms?

Breaking point

This tension can be found in the conclusion of an excellent monograph on the subject of queer theory and psychoanalysis. Javier Saez questions the progressist declarations of a resolutely Freudian psychoanalyst, member of the renowned *International Psychoanalytical Association* (IPA). Ralph Roughton, relatively recently, was delighted to recognize "the undeniable existence of healthy and mature homosexual men and woman."[29] Saez seizes hold of each of the terms in this declaration in order to illustrate the fundamental ambiguity. On one hand, it is indicative of a relative advance in the depathologization of homosexuality. In this declaration we could even read a real intention of opening up analytic practice to homosexual therapists. Such progress is a result of the prolonged struggles undertaken by some American psychoanalysts who came out of the closet and militantly worked in favour of the communitarian acceptation of homosexual subjects.[30] On the other hand, how can one not be surprised by the profoundly moralizing character of the conditions of this acceptation: "a mature and healthy life." Once again, we ask: based on what criteria? On what practices? According to what forms of love and relations can such a way of life be determined? And who is the psychoanalyst capable of making such a judgement?

Saez concludes that an insurmountable breaking point between queer theory and queer communities and psychoanalysis exists: "Queer theory questions the founding principles of psychoanalysis, such that it is not possible for *queer* to be co-opted by psychoanalysis as a complement or an improvement: we do not speak of the same reality."[31] With a decidedly queer irony, he turns the metapsychological vocabulary that is commonly used to refer to homosexuality against psychoanalysis itself:

> Are psychoanalysts qualified to be *queer*? Probably not. We could speak of the immaturity of their heterosexist manner of approaching the problem, of their incapacity to consider sexual difference, of a precocious delay in the development of sexual difference, of an infantile libidinal fixation concerning the phallus, of their insistence on reading gender performance in terms of structures or psychical realities.[32]

The author perceives a complete and utter incompatibility between the categories of thought foregrounded by queer theorists and the queer community, and those of analysts. In the closing lines of his monograph, Saez conceives of *queer* as "an Achilles high heel of psychoanalysis" on account of the position of the very "pronouncements of psychoanalysis."[33]

In a more radical manner even, Didier Éribon, whose antipsychoanalytic condemnations we have already encountered, has made himself the champion of the designation of psychoanalysis as a homophobic practice. According to him, the specialist of the unconscious dispossesses the oppressed subject of his lived experience, where the oppressed subject can be read as gays, lesbians, trans or queer. For Éribon, "psychoanalysis can no longer usurp the right to speak of homosexuality and take homosexuals as objects of study and of discourse without henceforth exposing itself to the return of the subject and their interrogation of this objectivization."[34] The advances in queer theory would correspond, as we have seen, to the ability of the latter to reappropriate such a consideration. Éribon asks

> Does psychoanalysis still have something to say to us, at a time of historic change where "minorities" have taken the floor in order to speak out and contest the institutions and the exclusions that they, the institutions, produce, setting about to invent alternate forms of relations between individuals, other forms of sociability, other ways of being oneself and of living with others?[35]

But Éribon goes further, He would like to definitively move away from psychoanalysis. He wants to settle the score once and for all. His work considers Lacan to be profoundly homophobic, where the latter would have liked to cure homosexuals of their ills, and who regretted the fall of the paternal order. By skillfully probing the texts of Lacan's seminar and his *Écrits*, Éribon shows to what degree Lacan developed, more or less unconsciously, a politically reactionary programme. "In Lacan, the questions posed in theory are drawn directly from the social problems in the contemporary world and his intellectual project explicitly presented itself as a political project."[36] Éribon drags Lacan back to what interests him as a historian of ideas: the sociological and political positions that must be deconstructed in order to transform the oppression of homosexualities into a source of pride.

If his work has the merit of forewarning us against an overly quick acceptance of Lacanian theory and even if his work has by and large contributed to both the destigmatization of homosexuality and the expression of the founding principles of a communitarian consideration of what it means to be gay, he nevertheless misses the heart of the matter as concerns Lacan's theoretic advances. Éribon expresses something of a fanatic hatred for psychoanalysis. His reasoning culminates in a pure and simple rejection: "All of this conceptualisation [...] that one would have to reject. What I mean to say is: psychoanalysis as a whole; psychoanalysis as it is."[37] He is so concerned with "bypassing psychoanalysis"[38] that he tends to forget what is at stake in the clinic and propels himself to transform Lacan into a monolithic block, oppressing all minorities with his transcendent weight.

Such a political project could be seen as being at work from the very beginning, in the publication of Lacan's first text on the subject of family complexes and could be seen to be little changed, regardless of the evolution of Lacan's thought: "The political function of psychoanalysis is to ensure the complete achievement of the heterosexual norm."[39] It is true that Éribon undertakes a meticulous reading: the carefully chosen excerpts from Lacan's writings are striking. And it is difficult to respond, justifying Lacan's statements concerning homosexuals in merely saying that they reflect a certain irony. Should one not just see a reflection of the times? Or should one subscribe to a portrait of Lacan as not being able to bear, even to the smallest degree, the "enigma of homosexuality?" Should one not see in psychoanalysis a mere "political and legislative instance of moral control, controlling ways of living, the arrangements that individuals construct in order to conduct their affective, amorous, sexual and familial existences as they wish or as they are able?"[40] To temper Éribon's anti-Lacanian hostility, it is useful to remind ourselves of the words of Élisabeth Roudinesco:

> Not only did Lacan agree to the analysis of homosexuals without ever pretending to re-educate them, or prevent them from becoming psychoanalysts if they so desired, but, when he founded the *École freudienne de Paris* (EFP) in 1964, he even accepted the principle of their integration, as *analystes de l'école* (AE) or as *analystes members de l'école* (AME). I myself was a member of the EFP and I can affirm that, in this matter, there was a terrific tolerance, even if, of course, many psychoanalysts detested homosexuals. "Private" and personal homophobia is one thing, the instauration of discriminatory rules is another.[41]

It is no less easy to depict Lacan as an utter homophobe. Éribon, in any case, succeeds in sketching a portrait of Lacan which is capable of discouraging anyone from beginning even a vaguely Lacanian analysis. But was it not already so with Freud? Could we not quite easily draw a portrait of Freud as fundamentally antiprogressive with a retrograde attachment to biology, to Oedipus and to castration?

Éribon's undertaking could seem unjust, or even insufferable, to a good number of analysts. It leaves no other choice, if we do not wish to "escape from psychoanalysis" or "be done with" Freud and Lacan, than to renew, not only the approach as concerns homosexualities, but also to carefully consider and show what advances the reappropriations, reformulations, and critiques that queer theorists and communitarians have aimed at psychoanalysis could possibly open up as concerns the study of the unconscious. Éribon's criticisms quite neatly confront analysts with the fact that free association – the founding principle of the analytic technique and the revolutionary foundation of Freud's enterprise – necessitates a capacity for listing within the context of transference which is open to even the most colourful differences. This framework of freedom cannot come about if analysts continue to act as guarantors for prejudices, age-worn refrains, and nondescript moralities.

Was Lacan gay friendly?

It is true that Lacan's irreverence is stinging to homosexuals, even if they were not his only targets. It is, in truth, difficult to excuse him. It is nevertheless necessary to see how Lacan's efforts notably permitted the renewal of the analytic practice in removing the weight of norms and morality. Lacan, through significatory listening, variable length sessions, the invention of graphs and mathemes, in locating jouissance or the Borromean knot, himself spent his life deconstructing a post-Freudian psychoanalysis which had been exclusively centred on the Oedipal, ccountertransference, feeling, the setting and which, little by little had lost its edge.

Lacan closes by situating the analyst in transference as a subject "supposed to know." In so doing, he admitted to not knowing the correct decision for the subject, in particular as concerns sexuality. As an aside, in his seminar on *Transference*, precisely where Didier Éribon reads striking insults directed at homosexuals,[42] Lacan does nothing less than sketch the contours of transference as a fundamental tool of psychoanalytic practice in using… homoeroticism. In fact, the seminar on transference establishes a rereading of Plato's *Symposium.* "It is certainly only insofar as he knows what desire is, but does not know what the particular subject with whom he is engaged in the analytic adventure desires, that he is well situated to contain within himself the object of that desire."[43] Lacan thus theorizes transference as a mechanism for the implementation of analytic speech as arising out of the love between two men. While it is true that he accumulated a series of coarse and sometimes bawdry allusions, the articulation of analytic speech could not have unfolded other than as a consequence of the Socratic experiment.

To summarise: Lacan was clumsy when he spoke of gays. Understood. And Freud, before him, reterritorialized, to cite Deleuze, the libido in the Oedipal. Well spotted. But, for all that, should we retain nothing from the analytic experience? From the moment when he who speaks lays claim to both his analytic practice and to his homosexuality as a point of departure from which to question the metapsychological whys and wherefores upon which the analytic encounter is constructed, the Achilles high heel of queer theory confronts psychoanalysis. We can thus ask, echoing Saez's metaphor, if the shoe fits?

Should we abandon the singular knowledge of which each subject is constituted, session after session, the distance that the subject takes on concerning the manner in which his life is interwoven, the benefits that he garners from this strange experience in which he opens up the most intimate fears and jouissance so as to uncover his desire? To attend analysis is to destroy the walls that oppressively hem us in so as to raise up the structure of our desire. To deny ourselves such a practice would be to deny ourselves a pathway to exercise our liberty. This is what the first rule of analysis invites us to do: "say whatever goes through your mind."[44] Éribon is right to underline the importance of the critical advances of communitarian ideologies. The latter do not wish for their desire to be dictated, they do not want to be cured in so far as they consider themselves to be neither deviant nor ill. In fact, they are not, no more or less than any other *parlêtre*. On the contrary, it is difficult to adhere to the substitution of the psychoanalytic process with "an analysis in terms of the stigmatization of one form of desire, and the social obligation, for the stigmatized, to act as if he were similar to others."[45] It does not amount to taking stigmatization into account, or to lessen the effects. Nor does it amount to being deaf to the communitarian claims for equal rights. Rather it amounts to realizing that, once equal rights have been obtained – and many struggles remain in this domain – the difficulty of being, of taking hold of one's desire, of knowing who one is and why, deserves to be uncovered according to a rhythm and pace that is strictly subjective, irreducible to any norm, unassimilable to any likeness, that is to say, following the rhythm and pace of a subject who advances and discovers themselves within the apparatus of the cure.[46]

Psychoanalysis should not be an instrument of normalization geared towards minor peoples.[47] It should not propose to heal them of anything at all but, more modestly, it should offer to listen, allowing the subject to explain their existence to themselves, not only in terms of sociological, ideological, or political determinants, not only in terms of the dominations and injustices which have marked their path, but in terms of the manner in which they have lived within their own bodies, allowing them to put words to these experiences. In other words, to see the implications of the marks that the Other (in terms of society, family, and language) has left upon his body, and understand their irreducibility.

Moreover, victory in struggles for equal rights for all, while necessary, is not enough to ensure happiness. If this were true it would be difficult to understand why so many privileged heterosexuals continue to wish to lie down upon the analyst's couch. Being within social norms, being a man, white, a member of the bourgeoisie, makes many aspects of life so much easier, but does not inoculate one from the weight of being. Of course, this does not amount to diminishing inequalities of gender, class, or race. But it amounts to reminding ourselves that no one, regardless of orientation or preference, is shielded from suffering, from the unsolvable blurring between body and language: fears, torments, wandering, and doubts when faced with the inevitable awareness of death.

On Achilles high heels

Forming one of the foundations for the queer project, Sedgwick remarks that gender itself appears as a category which arises out of ambient heteronormativity. She is surprised at the abatement of the multiplicity of sexual pleasures that is thereby undertaken. Irremediably, the topographies of erotic pleasure and of sexual acts are reduced to the classic oppositions that characterise the 20th century: homo/heterosexual, man *or* woman.[48] She concludes that "a great deal depends – for all women, for lesbians, for gay men and possibly for all men – on the fostering of our ability to arrive at an understanding of sexuality that will respect a certain irreducibility in it to the terms and relations of gender."[49]

This accounting for that which is most singular opens up a space for a possible encounter between a resolutely post-Oedipal psychoanalysis and queer theory.[50] From the point of view of speaking bodies, does the plasticity of the drives,[51] and the incoherence of jouissance not refer back to both the identitarian deregistration and the detonation of normalized identity as practiced by queer theory?[52] Localizing the jouissance of the subject, establishing its genealogy, envisioning how to live with it, encountering everyone on a case-by-case basis is not far from a willingness to see how "sexuality extends along so many dimensions that aren't well-described in terms of the gender of object-choice at all."[53]

Without falling into naïve optimism of an undefined reconciliation, those who are comfortable with their sexuality as well as with their desire, have a duty to share their experiences. For the misunderstanding between gender and desire,[54] if simply avoided, is at risk of perpetuating itself. And thus, without ever succeeding in bridging the gap which singularizes these spaces where we do not speak in order to make ourselves understood by the other, but where we speak in order to hear what is said (*le Dire*).

Anyone who experiences analysis knows that his words are not *analysed* but that rather, they are returned to him as *analysand*. Heterosexual, homosexual, bi, trans, the clinical experience does not exist in order to merely box the subject in theoretically, but in order to learn something about his singularity and to allow the subject to understand it. The position of psychoanalysis is not a position of knowing, but of surprise. The analyst is there so that the subject can seize upon the whys and wherefores of his "subjective *bricolage*"[55]: that which permits him to hold on, and that onto which he holds. Nonetheless, those who are homosexual experience, on a daily basis, the necessity of putting an end to the dirty little secret, the demands of fighting for recognition and for acceptance of the singular banality of their modes of loving and of enjoyment. Make no mistake, the subject of the drive does not erase itself, it ex-sists relative to the discourse in which each subjectivity is shaped. The rolling gait of one who moves forward on Achilles high heels arises out of that precarious cohabitation of a driven subject that ex-sists together with an engaged subjectivity that re-sists.

Queer theorists, queer individuals, speak to the analyst when they invite him to reflect upon the implicit referents which underpin his practice. They take him by the hand, show him that if he needs to embrace abnormality in order to grasp desire, he should nevertheless remain watchful so as to spot the violence with which norms are imposed upon the subjects that he encounters. The post-communitarian thought and demands of restive subjectivities do not end at the doors of the practice. They redraw the contours of the analytic relationship, intimately reconnecting it to its very foundation: speech and silence. Without a doubt, the analytic practice, more than a mere closet, thus closely resembles the famous chimney that Anna O.[56] referenced – and from which nobody emerges without being soiled. If the dirty little secret has no reason for being in the aforementioned spaces, well then neither does purity: grime and tears, eroticism and pain, words and bodies.

Emerging from the chimney

The chimney flue is one of the most obvious sexual metaphors. There is a Jewish story: two men emerge from a chimney flue, one clean and one dirty. How is that possible, asks the Rabbi. It is worth noting that the chimney sweeps are both men, cramped, in a small flue that pushes them one against the other. If the punchline of the story testifies to the absurdity of the question: has one ever seen two men, emerge from the same chimney flue, where one is covered in soot and the other not? This illustrates the way in which the analyst has a role and a function to play, but that all is not quite that simple. The analyst can play the role, but not without sticking their neck out, not without inconveniencing themselves. The considerations relating to transference and countertransference are illustrated by the profoundly (homo-)sexual character of this anecdote, and this allows us to review these concepts dispelling any hint of homophobia. Let us take a look.

From his very first accounts, Freud only spoke of transference in one direction: from the patient (female) towards their analyst (male). Think of Dora, think of Sidonie, think of the fuss surrounding Anna O.'s false pregnancy during her analysis with Breuer.[57] Even though Freud seems to condemn countertransference, that is to say that which the analyst feels for his patient, in order to favour the patient's discourse, the mention of countertransference is nevertheless tempered by a manifest heterosexism.[58] The person effecting the cure is, first and foremost, a man, and the person being cured is a woman, generally in search of a father figure. Do we need to remind ourselves that psychoanalysis is built upon the practice of men who listen to women who are unwell? The spectre of the homo-analyst thus quite immediately disturbs the givens in a historical sense.

The young female homosexual and Dora answered Freud in the terms of his countertransference. In one case, as in the other, the father of psychoanalysis was overly self-identified in his role. It is striking to note how transference was not able to foster the full benefits of the patient's speech in these two cases where their homosexuality was either explicitly asserted or was the "strongest unconscious current in their mental life."[59] Freud was not able to truly understand the homosexuality of his patients, or more precisely the position that he embodied caused them to flee.[60] It is as if the structure of Freudian thought stumbled when women's desire was no longer polarized in the direction of a heterosexual object choice. This is quite clearly structured in his consideration of transference and countertransference as a driver of the process of the cure.

> The analyst must never under any circumstances accept or return the tender feelings that are offered him: that, instead, he must consider that the time has come for him to put before the woman who is in love with him the demand of social morality and the necessity for renunciation, and to succeed in making her give up her desires, and, having surmounted the animal side of her self, go on with the work of analysis.[61]

Without a shadow of a doubt: the analyst is a man, and the patient is a woman. And what is at play between them has a strictly heterosexual colour to it. This is how the path of transference is initially expressed, together with the first warnings against countertransference and the failure of Freud in both of these famous cases, both of whom were not particularly settled on the question of their heterosexuality, is clearer still. For Lacan, countertransference amounted to the sum total of the analyst's biases.[62] That which prevents the smooth proceeding of the cure is, for a start, situated, not within the analysand, but rather, within the person behind him. That which hinders the dialectic does not always stem from where we expect. And Lacan recognized in women the capacity to move themselves within the context of transferential questions...[63]

Homo-analysts?

The homo-analyst is supposed to know as much as the analyst. He knows no more and no less about the subject. He is *supposed* to. He is unaware of that which the person he receives has to say, to discover, to accept. He knows nothing of what the subject has to tell him. He quite simply assumes the function. But his manner of performing this role will be different from that of a Father. Out of the closet, his actions will be illustrative of the fact that his desire has cast aside the morality of the Father and its associated *straight erothics*. In doing so one is not, however, by any means exempt from prejudice. Nor is one secure from countertransference. Nevertheless, his manner of making the practice minor, consists of rendering possible, audible, speech as it has been traumatized by dominant language. Such an exercise offers support to a modality of enunciation that is capable of understanding and of listening, without short-circuiting, the violence and the weight of social and moral condemnation, as well as the reality of injustice and the necessity of the struggle. The homo-analyst knows not only the rules of analysis, but also the weight of discrimination. Let us underline once more that if, on one hand, the subject ex-sists, on the other hand, subjectivities fight back, they re-sist. If transference and countertransference have something to do with love and desire, it is something that they concretize in words and through writing, that which "doesn't stop not being written," that is to say: that which impedes all finality, any closing off so that always and forever anything that is possible may come about. The analyst is thus bound to be beyond the norms, as close as possible to the truth of his desire and his desire for truth which propels the cure. Capable of catching, mid-flight, the signifiers which underpin the jouissance of the subject to which he lends his ears. This calls for silence, non-action, a taste for evenly suspended attention: silencing oneself in order to be heard.

But silence and attention should not be confused with inaction. One takes part in the struggle; one participates in the awakening of the subject. This is only possible on condition that one is wary of the conditions required by silence and the use of words. Linguistic rules too often end up essentializing the heterosexual norm, passing themselves off as the primary and inevitable law. Being wary of this tie to language, is to refuse to hypostatize the heterosexual relation as a point of departure and of arrival.

Presenting oneself as a homo-analyst – but I am expressing myself badly, one should rather present oneself as a *queer*-analyst or as an analyst in a minor key, so as to sound out the plurality of possible reappropriations – signifies thus rejecting the presuppositions of discursive practices which have been subdued by phallogocentrism. Nevertheless, such a declaration, midway between the personal and the political, should not add grist to the mill of Foucauldian warnings regarding a biopolitical use of sexuality.

To say that one is an analyst and a homosexual, or queer, or trans, should, at the dawn of the 21st century, not be limited to an autodeclarative or autoidentificatory practice, to a presentation of oneself as proper or improper, audacious, or simply banal. At risk is one's inscription in the apparatus of sexuality only to reinforce the most normative aspects thereof. It is not a mere question or personal indiscretion. Nor is it a question of a simple choice, a personal preference, which allows one to better describe oneself. Nor is it an addendum, a supplement to speech, a final confession, a really good one that can be made, and which expresses more than could ever be said regarding the channelling of sexualities.

The declaration of homo-analysis builds on performative practices. It benefits from *queer* irony. It plays with reappropriation. It interweaves reformulation. It develops a capacity for action. It opts for strategic *empowerment.* It blurs the line between what can and cannot be said. It defies the rules of enunciation. It modulates the discourse in another fashion, sidestepping the transcendence of the phallic order. It unsettles the enunciative logic. It dislodges the roles and the positions of those who have the authority to decide what can be said, what can be formulated and what is audible. It exercises a "performative contradiction."[64]

The space that the homo-analyst occupies on coming out of the closet is that of a reminder. First, the analyst expresses his or her homosexual desire. The analyst affirms their enviable banality. Homosexuality is thereby described as just another form of desire. Its specific hue, its militant nuance, is less a psychological explanation than it is political. Radically, this declaration wipes institutions, colleagues, and the analyst him or her-self, clean of any lingering doubt of homophobia. It has been said. In analysis, is it not better for each and every one to take responsibility for their speech, whatever the content or orientation? From the outside, this performative act drives home to what degree the "erotics of passage,"[65] which the interior space of the cure represents, can never be polarized in a heterosexual manner. The fantasies that are revealed therein by means of the dream, symptoms, or parapraxis, can all find expression without having to deploy any heterosexual complementarity, regardless of the orientation of the person directing the cure.

Given these conditions, it is possible that the *talking cure* mutates. It would claim to be much more than merely *gay friendy*: not merely tolerating gays, lesbians, queers, trans, and transgender, but being able to put the singularity of their way of life and their manner of saying and doing into perspective, be it from behind or upon the couch. Recognizing the value of what we are and what we can become. Under these circumstances, working with the unconscious would benefit not only from the cutting edge that is specific to the unconscious itself, but also from deeply diversified and resolutely contemporary forms of friendship,[66] ways of loving, means of enjoyment, and forms of suffering.

Outside communitarianism

Do the claims of the homo-analyst not also consist of an appeal to a psychological truth? Saying "I am an analyst" and "I am a faggot" do not signify anything if these declarations do not twist and interweave among themselves. For as long as they follow each the other along the Mobius band through which desire is articulated, the repartitions remain stable. However, in following one we come to the other, thus the psychoanalytic impetus leads to the homosexual drive, and vice versa. The two communities meet, are interwoven and pass each other by. On the one hand, the analyst stakes a claim in social and psychological respects: "You have told me that you are homosexual, but you have told me nothing of yourself." The analyst is searching for the subject. His words surprise him. On the other hand, coming out of the closet drags the apparatus of the cure towards the micropolitical. One has to take the risk of considering the impact of this preliminary declaration upon the practice and upon transference. When faced with such a declaration, it is not enough to say that one is not homophobic. It is rather a question of being able to perceive how this difference, this detail, this orientation are capable of shifting the viewpoint of the analyst. This leads the cure to the necessary organization of "practices of heterosexist resistance."[67]

When Eric Fassin considers the effects of coming out, he remarks how these effects, even if they have a real personal repercussion, fall to a greater degree within the scope of a "politics and not [within] the truth of homosexuality. As a consequence, we would like to underline the fact that this metaphor [of coming out of the closet] is inscribed within a rhetoric that we can judge pragmatically with regards to its effects and not its truth. Furthermore, as we are in the political register, we are required to embrace a strategic mindset."[68] The homo-analyst, the queer-analyst or the trans-analyst, in coming out of the closet publicly, do not only want us to recognize the specificity of their desire. They attempt to redraw the contours of the chimney and of the consequent chimney sweepings. It is not a case of simply liberating oneself from the box that is at once oppressive and which precludes one from freely expressing oneself, rather it is to show to what degree the very existence of this box is indicative of a hierarchy and of inequality in the treatment of sexualities and in accounting for their modes of enjoyment. To make the performance of homo-analysis heard, is to offer oneself the occasion to thoroughly reflect upon the implications of coming out of the closet.

This posture reopens the ethics of psychoanalysis. It no longer condemns the *praxis* from a communitarian point of view, quite the contrary. Foucault wrote *The History of Sexuality* in order to explain the social and political construction of desire and of pleasure.[69] This history does not constrain us into casting the hypothesis of the unconscious by the wayside. The historic analysis of sexuality and of homosexuality recounts the creation of a concept. The constitution, at a given time, of a category of perception and repartition of certain practices between men and women. These frameworks of categorization were often used as a means of stigmatization. They were used to classify, set aside, delineate, and also to define, what was normal and healthy and what was not. For Foucault, or Sedgwick, the homosexual does not exist in and of himself, he has no stable identity, no essence. When we map out this character, the links between bodies and pleasures in their political, economic, medical, literary and artistic aspects become apparent. Of course, in their work these authors do not seek to deny the existence of homosexual practices before the 19th century. Their focus is on discussing the self-evident nature of this bipartition which, even today, seems so natural. The opposition between homo and heterosexuality, and its stronghold on our sexuality, did, perhaps, not always exist. Or even, sex may not have always been defined in the way that it has been in the wake of Freud. To quote Foucault:

> Is "sex" really the anchorage point that supports the manifestations of sexuality, or is it not rather a complex idea that was formed inside the deployment of sexuality? In any case, one could show how this idea of

> sex took form in the different strategies of power and the definite role it played therein.[70]

The constructionist advances thus dismantle any fixed conception of sex. They undermine any approach that would reify the relations between bodies, any universalist categorization. They do not, by any means, overlook the deviations, condemnations, and exclusions throughout the course of history. At bottom, the more the image and the precise contours of one, single, sexuality, divided between homo and hetero, disappear, the more the condemned margins, the disavowed minorities make their presence known. If the established order continues its ceaseless mutations, those who inhabit the margins, the transgressors, also undergo continual transformation. At every step in history, the appearance of order and of transgression changes: the univocality of the sexual is always affirmed in a different manner, and the resistances to this affirmation are always plural. Indeed, the subject of the unconscious is embedded within this tension. In this decorrelated locus, composed of a permanent dialectic between the self (Ego) and the Other (be it social, cultural, familial, or linguistic), in this bevy of transgressions, of excess, of inversions, of decorrelation between what the subject does and what the subject says, the minor ethics of the analytical apparatus intervenes.

The performance of the homo-analyst arises in the discomfort of a gap where psychological and communitarian consistencies fade away. According to Lacan, the position of the analyst in the undertaking of the cure is that of "the dummy [le mort]."[71] "The analyst would have to strip the narcissistic image of his own ego of all the forms of desire by which that image has been constituted, reducing it to the only face that sustains it behind their masks: the face of the absolute master, death."[72] Queerness breaks apart identities and rejects the mirage of a homosexual psychology so as to better grasp the impossible foundation of one, one single, community and to always and everywhere make the voices of minorities heard in their plurality. On both sides, the real of the death drive shatters the mirage of shared meaning.

Clinical modesty

Reconnecting with a gay friendly Freud signifies, without a doubt, being able to perceive within his text the glimmer of something that lies beyond Oedipal constructions. Reconsider the history of his texts. This means also understanding how Lacan's "return to Freud" cannot merely be reduced to an appeal to the all-powerful symbolic but consists, on a greater scale, of the suspension of signification, and an erosion of the excess of imaginary meaning.[73] In other words, instead of limiting oneself to searching for the reign of the order of the Father, it is better to scrutinize analysis so as to detect its minoritarian dimension. This, at the risk of reading authors against themselves.

Freud: "One must remember that normal sexuality too depends upon a restriction on the choice of object. In general, to undertake to convert a fully developed homosexual into a heterosexual does not offer much more prospect of success than the reverse, except that for good practical reasons the latter is never attempted."[74] To this case of "the psychogenesis of homosexuality in a woman" we can, at the very least, add two other relatively famous cases. Let us begin, for example, by remembering the note that can be found in *Three Essays on Sexuality*: "Thus from the point of view of psycho-analysis the exclusive sexual interest felt by men for women is also a problem that needs elucidating and is not a self-evident fact based upon an attraction that is ultimately of a chemical nature."[75] In response to suspicions of homophobia, here Freud questions heterosexuality to the same degree as homosexuality. On one side, as on the other, an enigma lies, something does not fit, something goes wrong. In fact, the wellspring of the *talking cure*, as we have seen, shatters the ideal of Reason by means of the plasticity of the drive, unmasking the "polymorphously perverse"[76] nature that is hidden within each human being. Elsewhere, Freud does not hesitate to affirm that "there is indeed something innate lying behind the perversions but that it is something innate in *everyone*."[77] The diagnostic category thus loses any pejorative connotation. It should rather be taken to mean, if we consider for a moment the Lacanian wordplay, a continual variation of the Oedipal: *père-versions*, to each his version of the father[78] – regardless of the genitor, the educator, man, woman, or other… From that point, the subject is determined, first and foremost by the pursuit of pleasure independent of his or her sexual orientation.

In opposition to the rightful anger of queer theorists and communities, and in opposition to the most ambitious gender deconstruction, let us remember that Freud, in 1905, affirmed that the drive had no innate attributes, and thus has no innate orientation other than the pursuit of its satisfaction. In lieu of biological evidence, the father of psychoanalysis favoured the emergence of an enigma. Rather than making strict use of diagnostic checkboxes, Freud enjoins us to lend an ear to the words of the subject in their vain attempts to discern, always and evermore, that upon which the subject falters in his encounter with the Other. Heard and refracted in the prism of jouissance and of desire, homosexuals, heterosexuals, queer, trans, everybody has to deal with the impossibility of sticking to the straight and narrow.

As an aside, in his letter to the mother of a young homosexual, written in 1935, Freud presents himself in quite a gay friendly light. The letter is, of course, well known. Freud writes: "homosexuality is assuredly no advantage, but it is nothing to be ashamed of, no vice, no degradation; it cannot be classified as an illness; we consider it to be a variation of the sexual function."[79] Further on he adds, "what analysis can do for your son runs in a different line. If he is unhappy, neurotic, torn by conflicts, inhibited in his social life analysis may bring him harmony, peace of mind, full efficiency, whether he remains homosexual or gets changed."[80]

This project whereby analysis could ensure peace of mind allows us to better situate the implications of psychoanalysis with regard to certain ideological claims that are proper to the field of queer theory. This is because psychoanalysis refuses any orthopaedics of speech or of the self, psychoanalysis is aware that the *parlêtre* [81] – that is to say the subject in so far as it is completely parasitized by language – will never find a discourse that is perfectly suitable.

Thus, psychoanalysis does not work at a given pace or through negation. There is no orthopaedics of the self in analysis. There are no valid norms. The fundamental inadequation between our bodies and language sets the rhythm of this enigmatic approach: no sublimation without failure. No utopia where joy and justice triumph. No naïve idealism wishing for the jubilation of fortunate souls, no civilization without war. Faced with unbearable existence, the Freudian proposition remains, in fact, relatively modest: to being the journey, limping towards peace of mind. This is cold comfort given civilizational struggles and injustices. Calling on each and every subject to mobilize themselves in the hope of harmony and peace of mind, despite the furies of the world and the culture in which the subject lives.[82] This does not imply laying down one's arms when faced with social injustice. The struggle for the validation of "sexual variations" rather than a morality of the sexual requires, without a doubt, militant investment. Nevertheless, according to the analytic hypothesis, militantism does not suffice in order to subjectively accept one's one variation of the sexual function. Justified and necessary though it may be, militant rage does not heal the rifts of subjective conflicts.

The voice of Sidonie, that of Dora, that of Leonardo, and of Michelangelo and those of all the cases of homosexuality who have been the subject of consideration in psychoanalytic and academic journals these many long years correspond to so many "conceptual personae."[83] Whether we hear their speech, their manner of expressing love to their lovers of either gender,[84] their dogs,[85] their work, or any other object for that matter. Their voices sound out in chorus. They intone that there is nothing condemnable therein. Nothing that would allow for the diagnosis of any arrest in the development of the personality. Their refrain unceasingly varies: it is composed of ways in which what Lacan terms the "ab-sense of sex"[86] can be faced. Connecting all these cases, hearing their multiple voices, is to sound out the polyphony of the analytic cure. Such voices constitute an "other space," a "heterotopia,"[87] to quote Foucault, a counter-space where each and every one can come and process, put words to that which is impossible to say, that which tears a hole in the intelligibility of their existence. What happens in these spaces, is an accounting of the outside-of-sense which animates each of our lives. Such a space defies neat and orderly constructions as well as understandings which operate in terms of the framework of the Same and the Universal, even defying the judgement of that which should be perceived as healthy or mature. The path towards a clinic in a minor key, post-Oedipal, in touch with jouissance, with case-by-case *nouage*, can be mapped out beginning with such a suspension of intelligibility: in this, we can see what the subject fundamentally lacks, we can perceive that onto which he holds, and that which permits him to hold on.

In extracting potential homophobic colorations from the analytic act, we can better understand the structural dimension of Sedgwick's remark: "I do not, myself, believe same-sex relationships are much more likely to be based on similarity than are cross-sex relationships."[88] Like any other, they must confront the beyond-sense and contribute the rough outline of their solution. In *Epistemology of the Closet*, Sedgwick underlines the links between language and the closet. It is not by accident that, after her long introduction, and before the chapter entitled "Epistemology of the Closet," the theoretician inserts a reproduction of the Oxford English Dictionary definition of the word "closet." Among the meanings that feature, one can note "*Skeleton in the closet (or cupboard)*: a private or concealed trouble in one's house or circumstances, ever present, and ever liable to come into view."[89]

Ironically, the closet, thus defined, appears as the space in which the real dimension of its death is inscribed in language. The lexicographic definition of the closet that Sedgwick proposes resituates bodies and their jouissance within their linguistic determination insofar as this is directly related to death. Speech touches upon the real. Coming out of the closet does not mean leaving the skeleton in the corner of the cabinet, but rather, it means making use of it as a framework for joy, for a gay life, in the light-hearted, carefree, and colourful sense.

Notes

1 Sigmund Freud, "The Psychogenesis of a Case of Homosexuality in a Woman" in *The Standard Edition of the Complete Psychological Works of Sigmund Freud*. Vol. XVIII. Edited by James Strachey, Anna Freud, and Angela Richards. (Hogarth Press, 1953 - 1974), 145–172.

2 See Editions érès. "Les homosexualités aujourd'hui: un défi pour la psychanalyse," *Cliniques méditerranéennes*, 65, (2002).

3 See Jacques-Alain Miller, "Des gays en analyse," *La Cause freudienne, Revue de psychanalyse*, 55 (2003).

4 See "L'inconscient homosexual," *La Cause freudienne, Revue de psychanalyse*, 37 (1997).

5 See Stella Harrison (ed.), *Elles ont choisi. Les homosexualités feminines* (Michèle, 2013).

6 See Hervé Castanet, *Homoanalysants. Des homosexuels en analyse* (Le Champ Freudien, 2013).

7 We should recall that it was only in the 1980s that homosexuality was no longer referred to as a "psychosexual disorder" in psychiatric manuals, with the 1987

reedition of the DSM III in the United States. In Europe, it was only in 1992 that the term "homosexuality" was removed from the illnesses listed in the International Statistical Classification of Diseases and Related Health Problems (ICD-10). For a more detailed history of the psychiatric consideration of homosexuality, see Malick Briki, *Psychiatrie et homosexualité. Lectures médicales et juridiques de l'homosexualité dans les sociétés occidentales de 1850 à nos jours* (Presses Universitaires de Franche-Compté, 2009). An excellent historical perspective can also be read in Sylvain Tousseul, "Petite histoire conceptuelle de l'homosexualité," *Psychologie Clinique et projective*, 22 (2016): 47–68.

8 This homophobic turn of phrase was used by the American army in order to sweep any discussion of homosexuality in the ranks under the rug up until the Obama presidency, being repealed by Barak Obama in 2011. Judith Butler proposes a particularly stimulating consideration of this solicitation to silence in Judith Butler,. *A Politics of the Performative* (Routledge, 1997), 103–127.

9 The recent publication by the French Psychoanalytic Association (AFP) of the journal issue entitled "La Liberté en Psychanalyse" represents a notable exception to the trend. In this journal we can read a historiography of Freud's positions regarding homosexuality, a bibliographic commentary of the depathologization of the practice as well as a translation of the round table that was held in May 2001 at the American Psychoanalytic Association conference and where three "gay" analysts discussed their training. See, "La Liberté en Psychanalyse," *Annuel de l'AFP*, 1 (2017). See also Michael Feldman, "Being Gay and Becoming a Psychoanalyst: Three Generations," *Journal of the American Psychoanalytic Association* 50, 3 (2002): 973–987. While these contributions are enlightening, they nevertheless testify to a strange silence.

10 Michel Foucault, *The History of Sexuality. Volume I: An Introduction*, trans. Robert Hurley (Pantheon Books, 1978).

11 Eve Kosofsky Sedgwick, *Epistemology of the Closet* (University of California Press, 1990), 42.

12 See Sabine Prokhoris, *Le sexe prescrit. La différence sexuelle en question* (Aubier, 2000). See also Sabine Prokhoris, "The Prescribed Sex" in *Contemporary French Feminism*, ed. Kelly Oliver and Lisa Walsh (Oxford University Press, 2004): 177–200.

13 Sabine Prokhoris, *Insaisissable Histoire de la psychanalyse*, (Presses Universitaires de France, 2014).

14 "Quant à ce qu'il en est, dans la pratique des associations psychanalytiques au-delà de la tolerance et des bonnes intentions, de l'admission de candidats à la formation, ou d'analystes members qui soient homosexuels et puissant le *dire* – transsexuels, à supposer que la situation se présente, n'en parons même pas –, silence prudent." Sabine Prokhoris, *Le sexe prescrit*, 6.

15 The pass is a procedure instituted by Lacan wherein an analyst testifies to the end of his analytic journey within three years of the latter's completion, sharing the insights gained with the psychoanalytic school. The school confers upon the analyst the title of "Analyste de l'Ecole," with the genitive understood as both subjective and objective.

16 Recently new, and particularly critical, readings of this case have been undertaken, following the publication of the memoirs of Freud's patient. See Ines Rieder and Diana Voigt, *The Story of Sidonie C.: Freud's Famous Case of "Female Homosexuality,"* trans. Jill Hannum and Ines Reider (Helena History Press, 2021). See also the remarkable work of Jean Allouch, *Ombre de ton chien* (EPEL, 2004) as well as the doctoral thesis by Marie-Paz Rodriguez, "De l'énigme au paradigm. La psychanalyse n'est pas homophobe," PhD diss., (Paris 8 University, 2015).

Furthermore, the psychoanalytic journal *Au loin l'oedipe, L'Unebévue* 33 (2015), offers several rereadings of specific cases.

17 This position is challenged by Anne Fausto-Sterling, *Sexing the Body. Gender Politics and the Construction of Sexuality* (Basic Books, 2000). We will return to this question in the final chapter.

18 Eve Kosofsky Sedgwick, *Epistemology of the Closet*, 53.

19 On the contrary, in the psychoanalytic field, as elsewhere, we never cease to recognize the excellence of a (heterosexual) couple who work together… As many banal, silent reminders of the habitual orientation of practitioners. Among numerous examples, we could cite Maria Torok and Nicolas Abraham, Rosine and Robert Lefort, Octave and Maud Manoni.

20 Eve Kosofsky Sedgwick, *Epistemology of the Closet*, 21.

21 Eve Kosofsky Sedgwick, *Epistemology of the Closet*, 48

22 To quote the performative logic developed by John L. Austin, *How to Do Things with Words* (Oxford University Press, 1962).

23 Eve Kosofsky Sedgwick, *Epistemology of the Closet*, 67.

24 Eve Kosofsky Sedgwick, *Epistemology of the Closet*, 24.

25 Sigmund Freud, "Leonardo Da Vinci and a Memory of his Childhood" in *The Standard Edition of the Complete Psychological Works of Sigmund Freud.* Vol. XI. Edited by James Strachey, Anna Freud, and Angela Richards. (Hogarth Press, 1953 - 1974), 98–99.

26 For a detailed perspective on homosexuality in Freud, one need only consult the thesis, as necessary as it is rigorous, of Lionel Le Corre, "L'Homosexualité de Freud. Première contribution à une anthropologie psychanalytique de l'homosexualité masculine," PhD Diss. (Paris 7, 2015). His thesis has also been published as a remarkable monograph, Lionel Le Corre, *L'Homosexualité de Freud* (Presses Universitaires de France, 2017).

27 To quote the eloquent expression coined by Maurice Merleu-Ponty in Maurice Merleu-Ponty, "Eye and Mind," in *The Primacy of Perception,* ed. James M. Edie and John Wild, trans. Carleton Dallery (Northwestern University Press, 1964), 160. Merleu-Ponty asked that the indifference of science resituate itself within reality and the opacity of things and of the world, following the example of painting.

28 Sigmund Freud, "Leonardo Da Vinci," 99.

29 "[…] l'existence indéniable de femmes et d'hommes homosexuels sains et mûrs." Javier Saez, *Théorie queer et psychanalyse* (EPEL, 2005), 136.

30 Regarding this point, consider the pioneering theoretical and militant work of the psychiatrist and psychoanalyst Richard A. Isay. His writing and his practice contributed to the depathologization of homosexuality from what we could quite easily refer to as a communitarian perspective. See, for instance, Richard A. Isay, *Being Homosexual. Gay Men and Their Development* (Farrer, Strauss & Girous, 1989). The perspective that I develop in this book however differs from his, notably as concerns the question of Lacan *and* the queer community.

31 "[…] la théorie *queer* questionne les fondements de la psychanalyse, de sorte qu'une récumération du *queer* par la psychanalyse n'est pas possible, comme complement ou amelioration: on ne parle pas d'une même réalité." Javier Saez, *Théorie queer et psychanalyse*, 136.

32 "Les psychanalystes sont-ils qualifies pour être *queer*? Probablement non. On pourrait parler de l'immaturité de leur façon hétérosexiste d'aborder le problème, de leur incapacité à penser la différence sexuelle, d'un retard précoce dans le développement de la différence sexuelle, d'une fixation libidinale infantile au phallus, de leur insistence à faire une lecture des performances de genre en termes

de structures ou de réalités psychiques." Javier Saez, *Théorie queer et psychanalyse*, 136.

33 "[...] haut talon d'achille de la psychanalyse," "énonciation de la psychanalyse." Javier Saez, *Théorie queer et psychanalyse*, 132.

34 "[...] la psychanalyse ne peut plus s'arroger le droitde parler de l'homosexualité et de prendre les comosexuels comme des objets de son regard et de son discours sans s'exposer, désormais, à ce que ces sujets ne viennent l'interroger sur cette observation." Didier Éribon, "L'insconscient des psychanalystes au miroir de l'homosexualité," *Psychanalyse que reste-t-il de nos amours? Revue de l'Université de Bruxelles* 2 (1999). Available at: http://didiereribon.blogspot.com/2007/09/linconscient-des-psychanalystes-au.html

35 "La psychanalyse a-t-elle encore quelque chose à nous dire, dans ce moment de boulversement historique où les 'minoritaires' ont pris la parole pour contester les institutions et les exclusions qu'elles produisent, et entrepris d'inventer d'autres forms de relations entre individus, d'autres modes de sociabilités, d'autres manières d'être soi-même et de vivre avec les autres?" Didier Éribon, *Une morale du minoritaire. Variation sur un theme de Jean Genet* (Champs/Essais, 2015), 220.

36 "Chez Lacan, les questions posées dans la théorie ressortissent directement aux problems sociaux du monde contemporain et son projet intellectual se présente explicitement comme un projet politique." Didier Éribon, *Une morale du minoritaire*, 266.

37 "C'est toute cette conceptualité [...] qu'il faudrait rejeter. Je veux dire: toute la psychanalyse; la psychanalyse en tant que telle." Didier Éribon, *Une morale du minoritaire*, 222.

38 "Le contournement de la psychanalyse" Didier Éribon, *Échapper à la psychanalyse* (Leo Schreer, 2005), 46.

39 "La fonction politique de la psychanalyse est d'assurer la pleine réalisation de la norme hétérosexuelle" Didier Éribon, *Une morale du minoritaire*, 269.

40 "[...] une instance politique et législative de contrôle des meours, des modes de vie, des arrangements que les individus construisent pour mener leurs existences affectives, amoureuses, sexuelles, familiales comme ils veulent ou comme ils le peuvent." Didier Éribon, *Une morale du minoritaire*, 216.

41 "Non seulement Lacan prit en analyse des homosexuels sans jamais pretender les rééduquer ni les empêcher de devenir psychanalystes s'ils le souhaitaient, mais, quand il fonda l'École freudienne de Paris (EEP) en 1964, il accepta le principe même de leur integration, en tant qu'analystes de l'école (AE) ou analystes membres de l'école (AME). J'ai moi-même été member de l'EFP et je peux affirmer qu'il existait à cet égard une formidable tolérence, même si, bien entendu, de nombreux psychanalystes détestaient les homosexuels. L'homophobie 'privée' et personnelle es tune chose, l'instauration des règles discriminatoires en est une autre." Élisabeth Roudinesco, "Psychanalyse et homosexualité: reflextions sur le désir pervers, l'injure et la contion paternelle," *Cliniques méditerranéennes* 65 (2002), 18.

42 See Didier Éribon, "Homophobie de Jacques Lacan 2" in *Une morale du minoritaire*, 243–275.

43 Jacques Lacan, *Transference. The Seminar of Jacques Lacan. Book VII 1960–1961*, ed. Jacques-Alain Miller, trans. Bruce Fink (Polity, 2015), 193.

44 Sigmund Freud, "On Beginning the Treatment (Further Recommendations on the Technique of Psycho-analysis I)" in *The Standard Edition of the Complete Psychological Works of Sigmund Freud*. Vol. XII. Edited by James Strachey, Anna Freud, and Angela Richards. (Hogarth Press, 1953 - 1974), 135.

45 "[…] une analyse en termes de stigmatisation d'un type de désir, et d'obligation sociale, pour le stigmatisé, de faire comme s'il était semblable aux autres." Didier Éribon, *Une morale du minoritaire*, 281.

46 See Jacques Lacan, "Logical Time and the Assertion of Anticipated Certainty" in *Écrits*, trans. Bruce Fink (W.W. Norton & Company, 2006), 161–175.

47 According to Foucault's criticism of psychoanalysis in Michel Foucault, *The History of Sexuality*. For a broader perspective on this aspect of Foucault's work and on its consequences for the gay community see also Didier Éribon excellent reading of this subject in Didier Éribon, *Insult and the Making of the Gay Self*, trans. Michael Lucey (Duke University Press, 2004).

48 These oppositions are, in fact, quite recent, as the works of Jonathan Ned Katz and Thomas Laqueur illustrate. See Jonathan Ned Katz, *The Invention of Heterosexuality* (Dutton, 1995) and Thomas Laqueur, *Making Sex. Body and Gender from the Greeks to Freud* (Harvard University Press, 1990).

49 Eve Kosofsky Sedgwick, *Epistemology of the Closet*, 16.

50 Which is what Tim Dean hints at in his article Tim Dean, "Lacan et la théorie *queer*," *Cliniques méditerranéennes* 74 (2006). See also Tim Dean, "Lacan and queer theory" in *The Cambridge Companion to Lacan*, ed. Jean-Michel Rabaté (Cambridge University Press, 2003), 238–252.

51 On the question of the drive and the place that it occupies in subjects inhabited by language see Sigmund Freud, "Instincts and their Vicissitudes" in *The Standard Edition of the Complete Psychological Works of Sigmund Freud*. Vol. XIV, 117–140.

52 As concerns this point, see Jacques-Alain Miller, "Des gays en analyse?" *La Cause freudienne, Revue de psychanalyse*, 55 (2003), 82–90. See also Javier Saez, *Théorie queer et psychanalyse*.

53 Eve Kosofsky Sedgwick, *Epistemology of the Closet*, 35.

54 Regarding this point see Vincent Bourseul, *Le sexe réinventé par le genre. Une construction psychanalytique* (ERES, 2016). His work illustrates how gender and psychoanalysis are not opposed to one another but how the former nourishes the latter and vice versa.

55 "[…] bricolage subjectif" to cite the reading of *The Savage Mind* by Claude Lévi-Strauss that Hervé Castanet offers in Hervé Castanet, *Homoanalysants*, 156.

56 Concerning this point, I recommend the enlightening work by Gloria Leff, *Portraits de femmes en analyse. Lacan et le contre-transfert* (EPEL, 2009). Leff takes up the words of Joseph Breuer's famous patient, Anna O., or Bertha Pappenheim, her true name, in order to situate transference and countertransference in a Lacanian perspective. According to Anna O., analysis is equivalent to a "chimney sweeping." See Josef Breuer and Sigmund Freud, "Studies on Hysteria" in *The Standard Edition of the Complete Psychological Works of Sigmund Freud*. Vol. II, 21.

57 Remember that psychoanalysis began with the case of "Anna O.," who developed symptoms of a false pregnancy following her treatment with Josef Breuer. Freud, for his part, named his daughter after his old friend's patient: Anna. Anna herself became a psychoanalyst, and a lesbian, without ever coming out of the closet. Concerning Anna Freud's homosexuality and her secret, see Philippe Lacadée, "Extirper sa libido du coin où elle s'est tapie" in Stella Harrison (ed.), *Elles ont choisi. Les homosexualités feminines.*

58 Heterosexism is not equivalent to homophobia. It is limited to a series of behaviours and representations that privilege sexuality as viewed through the heterosexual prism, which accords it superiority as compared to other types and forms of sexuality. This point is developed in the following chapter.

59 Sigmund Freud, "Fragment of an analysis of a Case of Hysteria" in *The Standard Edition of the Complete Psychological Works of Sigmund Freud.* Vol. VII, 120.
60 Regarding this see the comments made by Sidonie Csillag several years after her encounter with Freud where she referred to him as a boor and as detestable. See Ines Rieder and Diana Voigt, *The Story of Sidonie C.: Freud's Famous Case of "Female Homosexuality."*
61 Sigmund Freud, "Observations on Transference-Love" in *The Standard Edition of the Complete Psychological Works of Sigmund Freud.* Vol. XII, 163.
62 Jacques Lacan, "The Function and Field of Speech and Language in Psychoanalysis" in *Écrits*, 252. On the subject of transference and countertransference in the context of the cure, see the work of Patrick Guyomard, whose work has largely inspired these pages. Patrick Guyomard (ed.), *Lacan et le contre-transfert* (Presses Universitaires de France, 2011).
63 See Jacques Lacan, *Anxiety. The Seminar of Jacques Lacan. Book X 1962–1963*, ed. Jacques-Alain Miller, trans. A.R. Price (Polity, 2014), 178, 183, and 197.
64 Judith Butler gives a precise definition of this term (which she uses to rethink the universal) in an interview: "The expression was used by Habermas to critique certain positions that he referred to as 'postmodern.' He was of the opinion that the critical claims made by the so-called postmodern positions could not be based on their own authority and that, in their articulation, they dismantled their own efficacity in offering no means by which their claims could be legitimised.

My interest is to understand how the framework or tables of validity were established, and whether a critique of these established frameworks of reference is, by definition, 'unfounded.' If one wants to critique conventional founding principles, one would thus be referred to as 'baseless' by those who occupy these foundations in an acritical manner. My hope is that it could be possible to, once again, seize upon the importance of critique and of critical theory over and above, and against, those who seek to establish a new foundationalism." / "L'expression a été utilisée par Habermas pour critiquer certaines positions qu'il appelle 'postmodernes.' Son avis est que les revendications critiques faites par les prétendues positions postmodernes ne peuvent pas se fonder elles-mêmes, et que dans leur énonciation, elles défont leur propre efficacité en n'offrant aucun moyen de légitimer leurs revendications.

Mon intérêt est de comprendre comment ont été établis les cadres ou les grilles de validité, et si une critique de ces cadres de référence établis est, par définition, 'infondée.' Si l'on veut critiquer des fondements conventionnels, on sera alors appelé 'infondé' par ceux qui occupent ces fondements de façon acritique. Mon espoir est qu'il soit possible de ressaisir l'importance de la critique et de la théorie critique par-dessus et contre ceux qui cherchent à établir un nouveau fondationnalisme." Judith Butler, "Vivre sa vie. Entretien avec Judith Butler" *Contretemps* 1 (2017). https://www.contretemps.eu/entretien-butler-subversion/
65 See Jean Allouch, *La Psychanalyse: une érotologie de passage* (EPEL, 1998).
66 As echoes in the title of Michel Foucault's brilliant interview. See Michel Foucault, "Friendship as a Way of Life" in *Ethics, Subjectivity and Truth: The Essential Works of Michel Foucault 1954–1984, Volume I*, ed. Paul Rabinow, trans. Robert Hurley and John Johnston (The New Press, 1997).
67 "[...] pratiques de résistances à l'hétérocentrism." Eric Fassin, *L'Inversion de la question homosexuelle* (Editions Amsterdam, 2008), 102.
68 "politique et non [dans] la verité de l'homosexualité. En conséquence, on voudrait souligner que cette métaphore [de la sortie du placard] s'inscrit dans une rhétorique qu'on jugera pragmatiquemen sur ses effets et non sur sa verité. Aussi,

puisque nous somes dans le register politique, nous faut-il entrer dans une logique stratégique." Eric Fassin, *L'Inversion de la question homosexuelle*, 98.
69 Michel Foucault, *The History of Sexuality. Volume I: An Introduction.*
70 Michel Foucault, *The History of Sexuality. Volume I: An Introduction*, 152.
71 Jacques Lacan, "The Direction of the Treatment and the Principles of Its Power" in *Écrits*, 492. For a detailed examination of the differences occurrences of the analyst as one who plays the role of the dummy [*le mort*] in Lacan's teaching see Patrick de Neuter, "Que doit être un désir du psychanalyste pour qu'il opère de façon correcte?" *Le Bulletin freudien. Association Lacanienne Internationale* 48 (2006). https://association-freudienne.be/wp-content/uploads/2023/11/44-07_De_Neuter.pdf
72 Jacques Lacan, "Variations on the Standard Treatment" in *Écrits*, 289.
73 Here, Lacan offers us a particularly useful indication, "Between centre and absence, between knowledge and jouissance, there is littoral which only turns to the literal insofar as this turn, you can take it in the same way at each and every moment. It is only through this that you can take yourself as the agent sustaining it." Jacques Lacan, "Lituraterre" trans. Dany Nobus, *Continental Philosophy Review* 46 (2013), 331–332. Thus, Lacan asserts the shift that is proper to interpretation: to no longer aim for meaning, norms, the plenitude of the subject that creates literature, but to aim at the letter. Lacan opens this text in remarking on the assonance between letter and litter. Interpretation must aim for this point where "the singularity of the hand crushes the universal," that is, the weight of the letter insofar as it shapes the subject in a radical and singular manner.
74 Sigmund Freud, "The Psychogenesis of a Case of Homosexuality in a Woman" in *The Standard Edition of the Complete Psychological Works of Sigmund Freud.* Vol. XVIII, 151.
75 Sigmund Freud, "Three Essays on the Theory of Sexuality" in *The Standard Edition of the Complete Psychological Works of Sigmund Freud.* Vol. VII, 146.
76 Sigmund Freud, "Three Essays on the Theory of Sexuality" in *The Standard Edition of the Complete Psychological Works of Sigmund Freud.* Vol. VII, 191.
77 Sigmund Freud, "Three Essays on the Theory of Sexuality" in *The Standard Edition of the Complete Psychological Works of Sigmund Freud.* Vol. VII, 171.
78 See Jacques Lacan, *R.S.I: Séminaire XXII 1974–1975*, ed. Henri Cesbron-Lavau (Éditions de l'Association Freudienne Internationale, 2002) Non-commercial publication. For further discussion of the teachings of Lacan concerning perversion see Hervé Castanet, *La Perversion* (Anthropos, 2012) and Franco Lolli, *Le Perversiono nella clinica psicoanalitica* (Poieisis, 2010).
79 Sigmund Freud, *The Letters of Sigmund Freud*, ed. Ernst L. Freud (Basic Books, 1975), 423.
80 Sigmund Freud, *The Letters of Sigmund Freud*, ed. Ernst L. Freud (Basic Books, 1975), 423–424.
81 Echoing the expression used by Lacan in "Joyce the Symptom," see Jacques Lacan, "Joyce the Symptom" in *The Sinthome. The Seminar of Jacques Lacan. Book XXIII 1975–1976*, ed. Jacques-Alain Miller, trans. A.R. Price (Polity, 2016), 141–148. For further perspectives in the birth of the concept see Colette Soler, "Du Parlêtre," *L'En-je lacanien* 11 (2008), 23–33.
82 See Sigmund Freud, "Civilization and its Discontents" in *The Standard Edition of the Complete Psychological Works of Sigmund Freud.* Vol. XXI, 64–148. See also Sigmund Freud, "Thoughts for the Times on War and Death" in *The Standard Edition of the Complete Psychological Works of Sigmund Freud.* Vol. XIV, 275–301. See furthermore, Sigmund Freud, "Why War?" in *The Standard Edition of the Complete Psychological Works of Sigmund Freud.* Vol. XXII, 197–218.

83 According to the expression used by Deleuze and Guattari, "the role of the conceptual personae is to show thought's territories, its absolute deterritorializations and reterritorializations." Gilles Deleuze and Félix Guattari, *What is Philosophy?* trans. Hugh Tomlinson and Graham Burcell (Columbia University Press, 1994), 69.
84 See Monique Wittig and Sande Zeig, *Lesbian Peoples, Material for a Dictionary* (Avon Books, 1979).
85 According to the hypotheses regarding the interpretation of the case of the young homosexual girl forwarded by Jean Allouch, *Ombre de ton chien* as well as those in the doctoral thesis by Marie-Paz Rodriguez, "De l'énigme au paradigm. La psychanalyse n'est pas homophobe," PhD diss., (Paris 8 University, 2015).
86 Concerning the ab-sense of sex One can only refer to Jacques Lacan, "L'Étourdit" in *Autres Ecrits* (Seuil, 2001), 449–496. Christian Fierens offers an enlightening reading of this difficult text in Christian Fierens, *Le Discours psychanalytique: une deuxième lecture de* L'Étourdit (ERES, 2012) as well as in Christian Fierens, *Lecture de* L'Étourdit. *Lacan 1972* (L'Harmattan, 2002). We will return to this concept in the closing chapter.
87 Michel Foucault, "Of Other Spaces," *Diacritics* 16, no. 1 (Spring 1986): 22–27.
88 Eve Kosofsky Sedgwick, *Epistemology of the Closet*, 159.
89 Eve Kosofsky Sedgwick, *Epistemology of the Closet*, 64.

Bibliography

Allouch, Jean. *La Psychanalyse: une érotologie de passage.* EPEL, 1998.

Allouch, Jean. *Ombre de ton chien.* EPEL, 2004.

Austin, John L. *How to Do Things with Words.* Oxford University Press, 1962.

Bourseul, Vincent. *Le sexe réinventé par le genre. Une construction psychanalytique.* ERES, 2016.

Briki, Malick. *Psychiatrie et homosexualité. Lectures médicales et juridiques de l'homosexualité dans les sociétés occidentales de 1850 à nos jours.* Presses Universitaires de Franche-Compté, 2009.

Butler, Judith. *Excitable Speech. A Politics of the Performative.* Routledge, 1997.

Butler, Judith. "Vivre sa vie. Entretien avec Judith Butler" *Contretemps* 1 (2017). https://www.contretemps.eu/entretien-butler-subversion/.

Castanet, Hervé. *La Perversion.* Anthropos, 2012.

Castanet, Hervé. *Homoanalysants. Des homosexuels en analyse.* Le Champ Freudien, 2013.

de Neuter, Patrick. "Que doit être un désir du psychanalyste pour qu'il opère de façon correcte?" *Le Bulletin freudien. Association Lacanienne Internationale* 48 (2006). https://association-freudienne.be/wp-content/uploads/2023/11/44-07_De_Neuter.pdf.

Dean, Tim. "Lacan and queer theory" in *The Cambridge Companion to Lacan.* Edited by Jean-Michel Rabaté. Cambridge University Press, 2003: 238–252.

Dean, Tim. "Lacan et la théorie *queer,*" *Cliniques méditerranéennes* 74 (2006).

Deleuze, Gilles and Félix Guattari. *What is Philosophy?* Translated by Hugh Tomlinson and Graham Burcell. Columbia University Press, 1994.

Editions érès. "Les homosexualités aujourd'hui: un défi pour la psychanalyse," *Cliniques méditerranéennes,* 65, (2002).

Éribon, Didier. "L'insconscient des psychanalystes au miroir de l'homosexualité," *Psychanalyse que reste-t-il de nos amours? Revue de l'Université de Bruxelles* 2 (1999).
Éribon, Didier. *Insult and the Making of the Gay Self.* Translated by Michael Lucey. Duke University Press, 2004.
Éribon, Didier. *Échapper à la psychanalyse.* Leo Schreer, 2005.
Éribon, Didier. *Une morale du minoritaire. Variation sur un theme de Jean Genet.* Champs/Essais, 2015.
Fassin, Eric. *L'Inversion de la question homosexuelle.* Editions Amsterdam, 2008.
Fierens, Christian. *Lecture de L'Étourdit: Lacan 1972.* L'Harmattan, 2002.
Fierens, Christian. *Le Discours psychanalytique: une deuxième lecture de L'Étourdit.* ERES, 2012.
Fausto-Sterling, Anne. *Sexing the Body. Gender Politics and the Construction of Sexuality.* Basic Books, 2000.
Feldman, Michael. "Being Gay and Becoming a Psychoanalyst: Three Generations," *Journal of the American Psychoanalytic Association* 50, 3 (2002): 973–987.
Foucault, Michel. *The History of Sexuality. Volume I: An Introduction.* Translated by Robert Hurley. Pantheon Books, 1978.
Foucault, Michel. "Of Other Spaces," *Diacritics* 16, 1 (Spring 1986): 22–27.
Foucault, M. "Friendship as a Way of Life." In *Ethics, Subjectivity and Truth: The Essential Works of Michel Foucault 1954–1984*, Volume I. Edited by Paul Rabinow. Translated by Robert Hurley and John Johnston. The New Press, 1997.
Freud, Sigmund. *The Standard Edition of the Complete Psychological Works of Sigmund Freud.* Edited by James Strachey, Anna Freud, and Angela Richards. Hogarth Press, 1953– 1974.
Freud, Sigmund. *The Letters of Sigmund Freud.* Edited by Ernst L. Freud. Basic Books, 1975.
Guyomard, Patrick (ed.). *Lacan et le contre-transfert.* Presses Universitaires de France, 2011.
Harrison, Stella (ed.). *Elles ont choisi. Les homosexualités feminines.* Michèle, 2013.
Isay, Richard A. *Being Homosexual. Gay Men and Their Development.* Farrer, Strauss & Girous, 1989.
Katz, Jonathan Ned. *The Invention of Heterosexuality.* Dutton, 1995.
Lacan, Jacques. *Autres Ecrits.* Seuil, 2001.
Lacan, Jacques. *R.S.I. Séminaire XXII 1974–1975*, ed. Henri Cesbron-Lavau. Éditions de l'Association Freudienne Internationale, 2002. Non-commercial publication.
Lacan, Jacques. *Écrits.* Translated by Bruce Fink. W.W. Norton & Company, 2006.
Lacan, Jacques. "Lituraterre," trans. Dany Nobus, *Continental Philosophy Review* 46 (2013): 327–334.
Lacan, Jacques. *Anxiety. The Seminar of Jacques Lacan. Book X 1962–1963.* Edited by Jacques-Alain Miller. Translated by A.R. Price. Polity, 2014.
Lacan, Jacques. *Transference. The Seminar of Jacques Lacan. Book VII 1960–1961.* Edited by Jacques-Alain Miller. Translated by Bruce Fink. Polity, 2015.
Lacan, Jacques. *The Sinthome. The Seminar of Jacques Lacan. Book XXIII 1975–1976* Edited by Jacques-Alain Miller. Translated by A.R. Price. Polity, 2016.
Laqueur, Thomas. *Making Sex. Body and Gender from the Greeks to Freud.* Harvard University Press, 1990.

Le Corre, Lionel. "*L'Homosexualité de Freud. Première contribution à une anthropologie psychanalytique de l'homosexualité masculine.*" PhD Diss. Paris 7, 2015.

Le Corre, Lionel. *L'Homosexualité de Freud.* Presses Universitaires de France, 2017.

Lolli, Franco. *Le Perversiono nella clinica psicoanalitica.* Poieisis, 2010.

Merleu-Ponty, Maurice. "Eye and Mind." In *The Primacy of Perception.* Edited by James M. Edie and John Wild. Translated by Carleton Dallery. Northwestern University Press, 1964.

Miller, Jacques-Alain. "Des gays en analyse?" *La Cause freudienne, Revue de psychanalyse,* 55 (2003).

Prokhoris, Sabine. *Le sexe prescrit. La différence sexuelle en question.* Aubier, 2000.

Prokhoris, Sabine. "The Prescribed Sex" in *Contemporary French Feminism.* Edited by Kelly Oliver and Lisa Walsh. Oxford University Press, 2004: 177–200.

Prokhoris, Sabine. *Insaisissable histoire de la psychanalyse.* Presses Universitaires de France, 2014.

Rieder, Ines and Diana Voigt. *The Story of Sidonie C.: Freud's Famous Case of "Female Homosexuality."* Translated by Jill Hannum and Ines Reider. Helena History Press, 2021.

Rodriguez, Marie-Paz. "*De l'énigme au paradigm. La psychanalyse n'est pas homophobe.*" PhD diss. Paris 8 University, 2015.

Roudinesco, Élisabeth. "Psychanalyse et homosexualité: reflextions sur le désir pervers, l'injure et la contion paternelle," *Cliniques méditerranéennes* 65 (2002).

Saez, Javier. *Théorie queer et psychanalyse.* EPEL, 2005.

Soler, Colette. "Du Parlêtre," *L'En-je lacanien* 11 (2008): 23–33.

Sedgwick, Eve Kosofsky. *Epistemology of the Closet.* University of California Press, 1990.

Tousseul, Sylvain. "Petite histoire conceptuelle de l'homosexualité," *Psychologie Clinique et projective,* 22 (2016): 47–68.

Wittig, Monique and Sande Zeig. *Lesbian Peoples, Material for a Dictionary.* Avon Books, 1979.

Chapter 4

Inverted Heterosexism

Fabrice Bourlez

Beyond a gay friendly post-Oedipal

In *Se dire lesbienne*, Natacha Chetcuti takes a fresh look at some of the advances in queer theory, paying particular attention to the work of Eve Kosofsky Sedgwick. She undertakes a series of interviews with women who identify themselves as lesbian. The sociologist thus underlines the importance of identification and of nomination in the social space.

> To call oneself lesbian (or gay) is a risk, it means taking the risk that, at any moment the recognition of sexual orientation may monopolize all of the senses and understanding as a whole, and thus define the individual in their entirety, even if this is but a small part of an individual's life.[1]

Even if such a declaration is necessary in order to fight shame, there is a great deal of risk that such identification can be reductive: "she's a dyke," "he's a faggot." Refusing such a stigmatized identity, is, moreover, to refuse forced invisibility: "Do what you like, but to hell with discretion!"[2]

Post-Oedipal psychoanalysis could perhaps be seen to begin in the space beyond the reductive nature of such identification. Identifying oneself as gay, lesbian, bi, trans, or queer, does not suffice within the structure of the cure. For this is no longer a problem. Or even, this is no longer something that is particularly interesting in this context. The stakes of identification in terms of a rallying cry for an ideal or for a cause are displaced toward the singularity of a *hystory*, that is, the subjective account that puts truth to the test in testifying to the manner in which language is tied to the body and to sexuality.[3] It is not a question of denying engagement in militant causes, nor is it a question of diminishing their necessity. For the analytic apparatus, the subject ex-sists in the *said* that "remains forgotten behind what is said in what is heard."[4] Upon the ruins of the famous Oedipus complex, the demarcations of the journey with the unconscious have changed. The order of the Father, the transcendence of the Law, well-meaning Morality have all shown signs of their own fragility. Their slow erosion does not however

DOI: 10.4324/9781003612735-4

sadden clinicians. It does not alarm them. This alteration has been duly noted.

Nevertheless, in order to remain coherent, the post-Oedipal has a duty to carry forth and take responsibility for not only its posture of openness, but also its theoretical underpinnings, even in the most extreme consequences thereof. It is necessary to take absolute responsibility for the deconstruction of the theoretical foundations upon which the enterprise has hitherto been constructed.

The post-Oedipal unconscious continues to (un-)set itself to work from the starting point of significatory ambivalence, failure, confusion, senselessness. The understanding of what is said is less easily triangulated than is the point from which the statement is made. What thus emerges for the subject is the resulting and impossible affiliation with one-self. Nevertheless, this precise and detailed approach regarding that which breaks with the continuity of our lives does not shy away from a supplementary effort: interweaving the threads of the Exterior and those of the political repercussions. The post-Oedipal dismantles the coherence of the established framework so as to propose another, less rigid, less inflexible, more welcoming or more malleable. So be it. But, in the final analysis, it is also about finding the courage to linger upon the manner in which this novel description is woven. Without this effort, the post-Oedipal ambition of closing in on the real, on a case-by-case basis, its thirst to welcome each and every one in their myriad differences, even the amenity of its silence always risks reintroducing that which has already been condemned by the sedimentation of the Oedipal.

To practice analysis in a minor key amounts to disturbing all of the prejudices that an analyst may hold. Encountering the contemporary without blissfully adhering to it. Sidestepping the manners in which the present can be experienced. Remaining vigilant. Maintaining a reflexive effort to hear the world in the way in which it is and in which it expresses itself. This vigilance is not only appropriate as concerns a homophobia that may be more or less latent within the analytic field. We have already addressed these questions in the previous chapter concerning the performance of the homo-analyst, underlining the lines of tension inherent in both the appeal to discretion and coming out of the closet. But such a performance is not sufficient. It is clear that what is at stake in the cure is no merely composed of what the analyst can sustain outside of him- or herself. A further step must be taken with regards to this micropolitical positioning and the resultant tributary stakes regarding transference.

The work of Natacha Chetcuti, which follows quite directly in the wake of the work of Sedgwick and Wittig, critiques the weight of the heterosexual epistemological privilege, "that is to say that the apparatus through which individuals conceive of themselves on the basis of a sexual majority, at the very least represented as such, in comparison to which homosexuality singularises itself all while isolating itself."[5] "Heterosexual epistemological privilege" is the synonym of what, together with Wittig, we earlier referred to as "*straight* thought." Many equivalent terms can be found: "heterosexual conceptual matrix," "obligatory heterosexuality," "heterosexism," "heterosexual system of thought," "heteronormativity." This semantic network points, in a non-exhaustive manner, at the manner in which thought, its reference points, its presuppositions, its universalisms, its doubts, its problems, all develop within *a priori* representations that, because they are never conceptualized, end up being conflated with heterosexuality and *the* difference between the sexes.

> And although it has been accepted in recent years that there is no such thing as nature, that everything is culture, there remains within that culture a core of nature which resists examination, a relationship excluded from the social in the analysis – a relationship whose characteristic is ineluctability in culture, as well as in nature, and which is the heterosexual relationship. I will call it the obligatory social relationship between "man" and "woman." [...] With its ineluctability as knowledge, as an obvious principle, as a given prior to any science, the straight mind develops a totalizing interpretation of history, social reality, culture, language, and all the subjective phenomena at the same time.[6]

Minority groups question the post-Oedipal perspective: in what measure is this epistemological privilege, despite a renewed and kindly attentiveness, still at work in our way of welcoming those who seek self-identification within our rooms, and in our way of caring for them within the bounds of our institutional practices? How is the analytic exercise shackled to this privilege, this matrix, this system? Does the analyst's coming out of the closet suffice in order to call this into question? Do those who hear, understand and accept his performance immediately expunge the *praxis* of its involvement in this heterocentric structure? Is psychoanalysis heteronormative? Does its attentiveness, and the ear that it lends, contribute to the reinforcement of heterosexism? Does its metapsychology belong to the realm of *straight thought*? How can it move away from this? When the tools of the psychoanalytic apparatus seek to teach how to function with jouissance on a case-by-case basis, when they delimit the singularity of the movements of the drive, do they avoid reinforcing the heterosexist structure? Not always.

Not being homophobic does not preclude one from being heteronormative. Not dreading homosexuals, queers, trans, and welcoming them in their diversity, hoping that each and every one can be fulfilled as they so desire, demonstrating a deep open-mindedness, abandoning perversion as the sole diagnostic reference when faced with the multiplicity of sexual practices, can all still favour, despite the best of efforts, a framework of thought wherein the whys and wherefores remain resolutely *straight*.

From an epistemological point of view, queer theorists have struggled in favour of the multiplicities at work in our lives and fight against that which supports a sole and unique way of thinking: there is no "for all," no universal shield that can be brandished, but in its place, a conscientious detonation of the authorized references, of the self-evident truths and certainties, of binary repetitions.[7] Going so far, should it be necessary, so as to strain the very communitarian plenitude of grammar, of spelling, and even of the self-evident logic that underscores reason. Thinking in a manner that situates itself is to displace knowledge beyond a centre that is shared by all so as to engage in thought from the standpoint of the partiality of the margins. Inverting dogmas, self-evidence, convictions. Breaking them up in the name of those that they oppress.

We have understood, when I call for a clinic in a minor key, that I am not content in merely defying these explicitly homophobic positions. I would like to shed light upon the latently homophobic register, that which, lurking in the shadows of the unthought, ceaselessly returns in the form of a "of course, I am not homophobic, but…" In the hollow of even the most enlightened discourse, insidiously, an "invisibilization of homophobia" sometimes persists.[8] I don't believe that in order to lift the veil on this residue of homophobia it is necessary to construct a tribunal of the expressible and the inexpressible, report on the twists and turns of their remarks, of their entanglement in intellectual shortcuts where homosexuality finds itself pulled back, once again, into the orbit of perversion. Rather, it amounts to inverting the preconceptions that continue to implicitly pathologize homosexuality. In short, if today it is good form to no longer be homophobic, it is nevertheless not unnecessary to interest oneself in the implicit that hangs over the orientation of discourse. As Claude Rabant illustrates, from an authentically Freudian approach, "pushing these things to their limit, we should show heterosexuality itself into this great communal edifice of perversion."[9] As we have seen, for Freud, heterosexuality corresponds to an equally serious problem as homosexuality. But, in this case, why, today still, is being a man or being a woman still envisaged, in three out of four examples, as being a heterosexual man or woman? Why, when we speak of a couple, do we so rapidly envisage a heterosexual couple? Why, when taking parenthood into account, do we waste no time in imagining a father and a mother? Why, when we discuss desire or jouissance in general, do we have the habit of envisaging our words, first and foremost, in accordance with directions, detours, and impasses that are resolutely heterosexual? The same can be said for a vast number of psychological and cultural subjects.

How to explain what is not an explicit or violent rejection of homosexuals, but rather the prevalence of one type of sexuality over another? Why does heterosexuality ultimately continue to maintain a monopoly on common sense accomplishment, to be the reference point in terms of behaviour or lifestyle? How is it that, despite the evident liberation of sexual mores to which psychoanalysis has contributed, the future, society, family, even meaning itself all receive free reign only in terms of heterosexuality, where all other forms of sexuality are asserted as an excess, or rupture.[10] When Gayle Rubin uncompromisingly takes hold of the political dimension of sex and the resultant forms of inequality and oppression, she arrives at the following assessment: "Modern Western societies appraise sex acts according to a hierarchical system of sexual value. Marital, reproductive heterosexuals are alone at the top of the erotic pyramid."[11] Her consideration seeks to critique the social conventions that authorize or condemn certain practices all while deconstructing the essentialism of sex: that is, the theorizations that see in sex nothing other than an immutable ahistorical force, without determination or social repercussions. Not without irony, she sketches the diagrams which are meant to represent the hierarchizations of sexual practices and their evaluation in registers as diverse as morality, religion, or psychiatry. Each of these schemas concludes in heterosexuality.

> This notion of a single ideal sexuality characterizes most systems of thought about sex. For religion, the ideal is procreative marriage. For psychology, it is mature heterosexuality. Although its content varies, the format of a single sexual standard is continually reconstituted within other rhetorical frameworks.[12]

Despite the best of intentions, heterosexism has infected the organization of our thought regarding sexualities and prevents us from creating a "pluralistic sexual ethics"[13] which is capable of making the diversity of genders and sexual practices welcome without recourse to the unique beacon of heterosexuality. As Eric Fassin quite simply sums up the question, "after all, sexism does not prevent us from loving women. In the same way, affection for homosexuals does not always, in France today, lead to demands for sexual equality…"[14] Such a demand implies remodulating the manner in which thought regarding sex is expressed. Our interest in *hystory* should not abolish the importance of historicization particularly as concerns the category of "heterosexuality" and the social stakes that are tied to it.

Rereading history

The queer challenge is thus at least two-fold. On the one hand, the sexual is liberated from a metaphysical attachment to the biological and to the psychological in order to illustrate the social apparatus. On the other hand, a theory and a politics is established which extols not only the defence of minorities and their inclusion in society as it is, but which also undermines the structure of the aforementioned society. And so, if needed, even going so far as to incarnate an impossible figure, an unbearable figure, going so far as to reject the reproductive and familial ideal, that of the future systematically envisioned as "our children's future." In the radical expression of the queer theorist Lee Edelman, this amounts to refuting the neutrality of "reproductive futurism,"

> terms that impose an ideological limit on political discourse as such, preserving in the process the absolute privilege of heteronormativity by rendering unthinkable, by casting outside the political domain, the possibility of a queer resistance to this organizing principle of communal relations.[15]

Of course, the author does not mean to hold back the reproduction of the species through an indeterminate queer militantism. Rather he seeks to profoundly question the universalizing spectre and the optimism of the creation of meaning which is completely and utterly orientated by the innocent figure of the child (to come), "*telos* of the social order" which relegates to silence those whose relations and love lives are ill adapted to the heterosexual reproductive model. In short, deconstructing heteronormativity shifts the horizon of the world considered through the innocence of the children of tomorrow, to a return to the polymorphous perverse child which Freud considered to be humanity's prerogative. Even the organization of the thought that would seek to undo heterosexism, epistemologically heterocentric privilege, must "recognize that this same disposition to perversions of every kind is a general and fundamental human characteristic."[16] This does not only result in a more friendly attitude towards that which deviates from the heterosexual norm, but also calls into question its epistemological and political importance over and above other forms of sexuality.

Taking the same view, *The Invention of Heterosexuality* by Jonathan Ned Katz offers a decisive and enlightening historic perspective. In compliance with queer calls to action, the author illustrates how the category of heterosexuality, far from being immutably transhistorical, was essentially devised and took shape in a remarkably short period of time.[17] What is taken to be an unsurpassable point, a self-evident truth that is ubiquitously shared – the necessary oppositional complementarity of two, and only two, sexes – in a number of debates and theoretical constructions, sees itself profoundly unsettled, thanks to this meticulous historical study. Katz evokes the "unstable, relative and historical status of an idea and a sexuality we usually assume were carved long ago in stone."[18] Armed with historical sources, he explains how, in a little less than a century, heterosexuality progressively became a form through which sex and jouissance were framed. But the very act of considering this category in terms of historical construction strikes at it from a contingent dimension. It aims a blow at the heart of the manner in which the category of heterosexuality determines the contents of our reflection. In a particularly Freudian manner, the author asserts that "Rarely do we focus for long on the riddle of heterosexuality—our gaze turns quickly to 'the problem of homosexuality.' The problem of heterosexuality resists problematizing as resolutely as several other peculiar ways of feeling, acting, speaking, and thinking."[19] More than a simple orientation in terms of object choice, heterosexuality admittedly organises the sexes and pleasure, but it does so only at a certain historical juncture: ours. In this historical and social reconstruction of our bodies and desires that begins at the end of the 19th century, Freud plays a decisive role. Once again, there are tworeadings, one in a major key, one in a minor key, which each pay homage to his work, each in their own and different way. One can consider the writings of the father of psychoanalysis to be one of the principal cogs in the machine that contributed to the stabilization of heterosexuality as an ideal.

> Freud functions as major modern maker of heterosexuality's ahistorical medical model and as subversive theorist of heterosexuality's social construction [...]. His theories provide the most complex support of heterosexual rule and important tools for challenging heterosexual dominion.[20]

Even if Freud defied Victorian morality, even if he liberated sexual desire from any obligations regarding the reproduction of the species, even if he pinpointed the polymorphous perversion inherent in each and every one of us, the psychoanalytic tradition and society as a whole used his work as a foundation in order to erect a monolith ensuring heterosexuality as the unsurpassable qualitative outcome. "While rebel Freud often devastatingly questions the idea of normal sexuality, conformist Freud was normal sexuality's prime mover. In this age of science worship, the word 'normal' replaced 'natural' as the term with which to conjure up a new heterosexual ethic."[21] Once seen as a historically contingent phenomenon, heterosexuality effectively loses all epistemological prestige as well as any explicative prerogative regarding personal undertakings. Let us now consider how to return to "rebel Freud" so as to reroute his heterosexist metapsychology.

Defining gender?

In this light, the contributions of Judith Butler are without a doubt among the most useful in resisting a conception of the individual that draws on a uniquely heterosexual matrix.

We have already seen the fundamental irony with which she redeploys the theoretical pomp and ceremony of psychoanalysis. Against Freud read in a major key, Butler plays the minority card. Can this manner of undercutting the psychanalytic episteme open hitherto unexpected and new paths for the psychoanalytic clinic? Regarding this, Butler has no real ambitions. Reflecting upon the questions of mourning and of melancholy – to which we will soon come – she modestly declares:

> I make no empirical claims, nor attempt a survey of current psychoanalytic scholarship on gender, sexuality, or melancholy. I want merely to suggest what I take to be some productive convergences between Freud's thinking on ungrieved and ungrievable loss and the predicament of living in a culture which can mourn the loss of homosexual attachment only with great difficulty.[22]

In considering the post-Oedipal in a minor key, my goal is not to study Butler's texts as a new manual of clinical psychology. But, like it or not, her "productive convergences" shed new light, through critique, on that which is at the heart of the psychoanalytic experience: the (ir)relatability of sex and meaning. It would, however, be contradictory to welcome subjects in their diversity if the metapsychological foundations with which we exercise our attentiveness remain affixed to a heteronormative unthought. With Butler, we work upon a genealogy of metapsychological concepts. With the unconscious forming the site of a veritable micropolitics.[23] Approaching the question of the clinic in a minor key thus keenly touches upon that which makes the analytic act possible.

In the second introduction that Butler wrote for the republication of *Gender Trouble* in 1999, she reaffirms having written her book in order to open up the field of possibilities in terms of gender and sexuality. "One might wonder what use 'opening up possibilities' finally is[?]"[24] With this rhetorical question, the philosopher directly specifies the manner in which she would like to distance herself from a potential heterocentrist *a priori*. In fact, this reaction, "one might wonder?" can only really be formulated by someone for whom living out their sexuality, their gender, their body, contributes, for better or worse, to the sphere of shared self-evidence. On the contrary, this opening up of possibilities, reveals itself to be of a burning necessity for those who have "understood what it is to live in the social world as what is 'impossible,' illegible, unrealizable, unreal, and illegitimate."[25]

In enjoining us to think together with these "impossibles," Butler does not pull us away from the clinic. On the contrary, she radicalizes the Freudian gesture which drew on the symptom in order to understand what is properly human.[26] In fact, for Freud, on one hand "these abnormalities will have drawn our attention to amalgamations which have been lost to view in the uniform behaviour of normal people"[27] and, on the other hand, "the sexual life of each one of us extends to a slight degree-now in this direction, now in that-beyond the narrow lines imposed as the standard of normality."[28] The encounters that are woven in analytic practice are, indeed, replete with anomalies, illegible stains, blind spots, and aberrations. To lend an ear to them, right up until their ultimate outcome, is to decentre the unthought that structures the knowledge drawn from the unconscious. What is more, the Butlerian approach disconnects the individuation of the symptom from the ideal of an understanding of a "normal" sexuality, were this sexuality to be considered, first and foremost as heterosexual. In starting out from the margins, without preoccupying oneself with any adequation between the subject at hand and normality, we can hobble certain key concepts of the Freudian unconscious so as to renew their efficiency.

Butler teaches us that being a man, or a woman is an exercise in complexity without any guarantee of success. In this way, she sketches a territory wherein the assurance of the masculine desire orientated towards the woman no longer constitutes an end in and of itself, nor does it constitute a waypoint, nor even a point of departure on the path of reflection. "Gender is the repeated stylization of the body, a set of repeated acts within a highly rigid regulatory frame that congeal over time to produce the appearance of substance, of a natural sort of being."[29] But, if one has to deal with "repetitions," even within the "rigid regulatory frame," and if what finally prevails is "appearance," this signifies that the immobility of being is not ineluctable and that the rigidity of the framework is more supple than it may at first appear. At the very least, evoking stylization prevents one from falling into strict determinism.

Instead of providing an unequivocal answer to the question "what is gender?" Butler undertakes a reversal that bears significant consequences: "gender is not to culture as sex is to nature; gender is also the discursive/cultural means by which 'sexed nature' or 'a natural sex' is produced."[30] Gender – the "male" or "female" checkbox – requires a naturalizing fiction. Traditionally, gender represents the constructed, learnt, social version of that which arises out of the anatomical distinction between the sexes.[31] *Gender Trouble* manhandles this representation which draws a straight line from nature to culture. Thus, does gender "as the cultural interpretation of sex" not always already structure our perception of natural sex? Butler perseveres: do we have the means to reach a "'prediscursive,' prior to culture, a politically neutral surface on which culture acts?"[32] If one follows this line of reasoning, taking the beacon of biological sex as the ultimate abutment of one's destiny, is, in reality, to submit oneself to the cultural edifice itself. Perceiving the truth of one's being through physical presuppositions where the natural proof could, just as easily, be nothing other than a myth, inaccessible without the help of cultural constructions which are always already hierarchized by gender itself. In short, an unverified hypothesis.[33]

Here gender does not trace the contours of biological binarism, it stirs them up. Gender has imposed itself as a manner in which to give them consistence forming an interpretative point of view which believes itself to be devoid of artificiality. In other words, there is no reification of gender through nature, likewise, there is no legitimization of the biological through gender. By overturning the classical perception of gender, in considering it not in terms of that which stems from sex but in terms of that which is foundational for perception, Butler insists on the manner in which the body itself, its own materiality, even its flesh[34] is always already a construction built out of norms, discourse, heritage, gestures, postures, ideals… So, the category, while regularly considered as binary (either man or woman), would not be any less re-modulable. What would the consequences of this deconstruction be for the psychoanalytic structure?

Inverting the trajectory that leads from nature to culture leaves the implicit points of reference hanging. Butler asks: "Is the breakdown of gender binaries, for instance, so monstrous, so frightening, that it must be held to be definitionally impossible and heuristically precluded from any effort to think gender?"[35]

Elsewhere in an interview she states:

> I think that the work on gender was and is concerned with figuring out how we're made by norms and conventions that precede us and that are larger than us, and also what possibilities of agency exist for us, of becoming different genders or becoming gendered differently, given how we are made. I've always been concerned to understand subjective agency, that is, the agency we have as persons, as both constrained by certain kinds of cultural forces but not determined by them, and also open to improvisation and malleability and repetition and change.[36]

This notion of "subjective agency" does not seem to me to be so far removed from what one experiences in the analytic trajectory where, with every step, we see that is it always possible to invest answers or alternatives when faced with the Other, familial destiny, or anamnestic coordinates that are imposed upon us. Developing a capacity for agency amounts to accepting one's subjective responsibility faced with what we experience. The responsibility should here be extended to the etymological sense of the term: what type of response am I able to give when faced with the Other? But the capacity for agency can apply to the dispositive of the cure itself: how can the militant speech, combative and dissenting, of minor people have repercussions on the foundations by which they are determined?

Nothing is even ontologically established: not even *the* difference between the sexes and even less the unique reference to the heterosexual norm. Nevertheless, Butler affirms, in a vary Lacanian manner:

> Every time that we try to reference the body, we make this reference through certain modes of description or through certain frameworks of reference, but, every time, we fail to reference: there is something that exceeds this act of referencing and which breaks down, within language itself, the effort of making a reference.[37]

The rationality at work in the promise of gender thus entails this constituent failure of an ideal correspondence between the body and words. Butler has no other goal than to show how our bodies can ceaselessly learn to relate to themselves in a different manner. Beyond *straight* logic, these accounts make new trajectories of thought and new modes of living possible, audible, and liveable.

Fr-oucault[38]

Let us review. Both Freud and Foucault shed light on the manner in which subjectivity is woven, that is to say: how the subject cannot be reduced to an entity that is closed upon itself, but is always being formed and constituted due to, and by means of, an alterity which inevitably precedes it and, in part, determines it.

We are politically *and* linguistically determined by the Other. The subjective dimension of our existences is elaborated by means of power and language, which represent the loci of our subjection (understood both as becoming a subject, a person, and in being subjected).

> Power is often cast as unequivocally external to the subject, something imposed against the subject's will. But if the very production of the subject and the formation of that will are the consequences of a primary subordination, then the vulnerability of the subject to a power not of its own making is unavoidable.[39]

But this approach to the subject is insufficient for Butler. A hitherto unseen relationship between Freud and Foucault needs to be established. Not without malice, Butler recalls that Foucault "is notoriously taciturn on the topic of the psyche"[40] In reality, more than notoriously taciturn, Foucault had what can at the very least be described as an ambiguous relationship to psychoanalysis, from the very outset.[41]

By revising the relationship that Foucault had with the psyche, Butler not only connects him to Freud, but she also relieves the queer movement, direct heirs to Foucault's legacy in the USA, from possibly becoming caught in an imaginary representation of identity. Freud's text counterbalances the plasticity of gender, of the body and of sex, according to which one would be free to alter one's identity at will, according to one's taste, colour, or circumstance. The possibility of envisaging gender like a piece of clothing that can be worn was introduced by *Gender Trouble.*[42] Subsequently, Butler has nevertheless nuanced that which could mean being confined to a sort of ultra-nominalist capitalist relativism where each and every one would define themselves without any regard to the Other.[43] Considered in terms of its relationship to power, the psyche, in fact, opens itself up to the movements of identity deconstruction and naturalism. But, in return, it is no less bounded, anchored, in the excess that is proper to the drives: it is a "recognition that the subject produced as continuous, visible, and located is nevertheless haunted by an inassimilable remainder, a melancholia that marks the limits of subjectivation."[44] Norms and power are thus immersed in the weight of jouissance, in the return of the same, in symptomatic repetition. Such that the impossible and unbearable face that is specific to the reality of the drive superposes itself upon the plasticity of pleasure. Within the psyche, the jouissance of the subject, that which interrupts, that which causes suffering, that which is striking in its redundance, binds itself to the aesthetic and to pleasure, to practices and becomings.[45] The work of Butler recalls to what degree Foucault's invitation to "conceive of sex without the law, and power without the king"[46] should not be translated into a festive invitation to enjoy and love without constraint. Foucault's thought is to be inscribed within the perimeter of the psyche such as Freud's advances have been able to delimit it.

Reading Freud with Foucault also allows for the unsticking of psychoanalysis from the temptation of a potential personalism or of a well-meaning psychologism where masculine and feminine could be considered to be principal and unsurpassable beacons. This disconnects the unconscious from all confusion with any questions of psychological intimacy. This avoids enclosing it by having exclusively taken the coordinates of the family and of the associated fantasy into account. The Butlerian double vision leads this consideration to embrace a supplementary level of complexity. In fact, in thinking between Freud and Foucault, we do not only give up on a conception of psychoanalysis and the psyche as personological equivalents. We do not only refuse to confound psychoanalysis with moral enforcement, nor do we limit ourselves by holding back the biopolitical deconstructions or by recalling the inevitable anchorage of the subject to a tough and immovable kernel – whether it be referred to as the social, the linguistic or the real. Rather we question, in their micropolitical valency, the concepts which allow for the study of the psyche itself.

Thinking *agency*

Butler is able to give consistence to this impossible psycho-political chiasmus through a notion that is as rich as it is untranslatable in French: *agency*. From one book to another the term is variably rendered: "agentivity," capacity for action, power to act… *Agency* is the attribute given to subject in so far as they are no longer perceived as individual units, gifted with will and self-control, but as a site at the crossroads of the intimate and the public, at the intersection of linguistic determination and the effects of power, a space where the possibilities of self-transformation and self-alteration are inscribed and where it is possible for the subject to shift their dependence regarding that which exists. *Agency* is the other side of consciousness, the call to freedom of an unconscious which acts. Butler, in reconsidering the epistemological foundations of subjectivity and the political dimension of the use of certain norms, invites the clinician to reflect on the inner workings which are foundational to his practice, in so far as the clinician offers consistence to the discourse of the unconscious, thanks to, or as a consequence of the function that the clinician serves with regards to the patient. Can the theory of *agency* of which Butler sketches the perspectives in the course of her work interrogate the apparatus, or even the direction of the cure? How does *agency* concern both the clinician and the patient in the dis-connection that is established between them by the intermediary of transference?

Butler's progress rests upon the following paradox: the alteration of the self – on account of the subjection that is specific to power – never leaves the games of power as they are. "Such a formulation suggests that in the act of opposing subordination, the subject reiterates its subjection (a notion shared by both psychoanalysis and Foucauldian accounts)."[47] But, as Butler hastens to clarify, this subjection is also capable of generating an effect, of shaking things up: it is also a capacity for action. "The subject is itself a site of this ambivalence in which the subject emerges both as the effect of a prior power and as the condition of possibility for a radically conditioned form of agency."[48] This form of action, while "radically conditioned," does not any less exceed power, nor does it constrain power to new configurations. If power produces the subject, it is to an equal degree overtaken by its production. "Exceeding is not escaping, and the subject exceeds precisely that to which it is bound."[49]

Agency such as Butler thematizes it, appears thus as a tangible point of departure for taking another look at the articulation of the psychoanalytic corpus while propping it up against the clinic in a minor key. *Agency* opens up the possibility of altering the way things are. It should not be taken as a utopian insurrection. For all that, it does not abandon the revolutionary cries. It accepts original fallibility.[50] *Agency* is at once the failure of the subject as master and possessor and is that which allows for the creation of a new humanity. In *Frames of War*, where the theoretician is preoccupied with a consideration of the violence of war which parallels the formation of the subject, she asks: "How do I live the violence of my formation? [...] In what sense can such violence be redirected, if it can? [...] Can one work with such formative violence against certain violent outcomes and thus undergo a shift in the iteration of violence?"[51] In one swift movement, she associates the redirection of violence, her subjective reappropriation, and the work of psychoanalysis. "As such, non-violence is a struggle, forming one of the ethical tasks of clinical psychoanalysis and of the psychoanalytic critique of culture."[52] In other words,

> The point is not to eradicate the conditions of one's own production, but only to assume responsibility for living a life that contests the determining power of that production; in other words, that makes good use of the iterability of the productive norms and, hence, of their fragility and transformability. The social conditions of my existence are never fully

willed by me, and there is no agency apart from such conditions and their unwilled effects.[53]

This knot which is tied between, on one hand that which constitutes us, despite ourselves, in violently oppressing us, that which determines us within a framework all while escaping us, and, on the other hand the movements of the permanent renegotiation of this framework and the involuntary effects point to the at once fragile and necessary site of our capacity to act as political subjects and as subjects of the unconscious.

The capacity to act is tightly woven into "vulnerability." The fallible being, the flaw, set us upon the path of another theoretical undertaking, political and clinical. If the examples of displacements that Butler offers (minority assemblies, *dye in, kiss in*, "Las Madres de la Plaza de Mayo" in Argentina, the outraged youth in Greece…) turn out to be explicitly political, they are not any less disconnected from the unconscious. To what degree does psychoanalysis give back to the subject their capacity for action? Is the vulnerability that characterizes the site of the subject from whence Butler advances her reconstruction of the political space not the self-same space upon which the cure, with modesty, relies session after session? Does the encounter of the patient with the clinician, the relation of one to the other, the dis-connection which gathers their existences together according to the fundamental rule of the analytic technique – "say whatever goes through your mind"[54] – not imply, in both directions, an accounting for, primarily and decisively, the profound human vulnerability, the tie that signifies our unwavering affiliation to something other than to ourselves? The site of the subject is constructed in the course of this subjection to the Other. This dependence confers to the smallest of gestures, to the shortest of words, a fundamental vulnerability that is torn away from any fantasy of completeness. Out of this flaw which marks the subject with incompleteness, out of this foundational vulnerability an authentic power to act can nevertheless be born: a desire. There are many ways in which one can express Lacan's famous adage according to which "unconscious desire is the Other's desire."[55]

Nonetheless, attention: *agency* is not a one-way street. It allows for an understanding of the manner in which the power relations which animate the therapeutic link are defined by vulnerability. It is true that the patient who comes to analysis, supposedly in order to be treated, could seem all the more subdued and vulnerable in so far as they are faced with another, supposedly there to treat them. The clinical relation must not avoid this paradox: the two are present only to reflect, both, each in their own manner, upon this original vulnerability. "That subjects are constituted in primary vulnerability does not exonerate the abuses they suffer; on the contrary, it makes all the more clear how fundamental the vulnerability can be."[56] The psychoanalytic cure is articulated around this "lack of being," to be understood as the Lacanian synonym of the incompleteness specific to subjects caught up in the snare of the signifier. Rereading this in terms of *agency* thrusts it closer to the interrogations of minor people: how to seize upon the analytic apparatus in order to make ourselves heard? How to reappropriate one's conceptual matrix so as to no longer suffer its expropriation? How to inverse the power dynamic at work in the study of the psyche? How can our own vulnerability become a source of resignification for the analytic apparatus itself?

Performative speech and the speech of the subject

Faced with the fecund promises of decentralization obtained through *agency*, the encounter with patients does not any less question the coherence of Butler's theoretical edifice. In the final analysis, does the rigour of her epistemological and political positions not fail the concrete clinical situation which refuses systematization such that the singularity of scattered speech may resound: the tiniest detail, the smallest of degradations, the guilt of the unsaid, the force of desire upon which a surreptitious laugh breaks? So frontally questioning Butler's clinic puts her thought to the test when faced with the disorder, the turmoil that propels the real of live subjects that experience the cure. Once again, in other words, and at a tipping point, how are clinicians – who must remember that "psychoanalysis is not a child of speculation"[57] in order to hear the discourse of the subject – able to modify their *praxis*, alter their ability to listen, transform their manner of interpretation, having read the texts of this American philosopher? To what degree are the theories of Butler, following the example of Freud and Lacan, sufficiently consistent so as to hear and understand the accounts of analysands in a new and original manner? And, inversely, are they sufficiently inconsistent so as to respond, in deferred action, to the logic that is particular to the accounts of each and every one? Let us clarify, at this juncture, the value that Butler accords speech in the construction of gender in order to better specify its repercussions on the analytic cure.

According to the philosopher, gender, a social and linguistic construction, is a performative construction: a speech act that brings into being that which it names. In this, the philosopher seizes upon, and reworks to her own ends, the theory of John Langshaw Austin, for whom the performative is a speech act that is distinguishable from a simple affirmation in so far as it accomplishes an action. For example, a judge who announces that "the session is open," a mayor who declares a couple to be "husband and wife." The speech act has, in these examples, concrete and real consequences.

While it is similar, performativity should not be confused with performance. Rather, it is the framework through which the subject is called into question. In fact, theatrical performance, or the much vaunted artistic performance, which has enjoyed renown in the field of fine arts since the 1970s cannot exist without the mediation of the aforementioned "performance," of the one who does what is in the process of being done…[58] However, Butler is interested, firstly, in the status of language, in its political, social, physical, and psychic impact. The performative clearly reveals uses of language that are detached from one or another personally incarnate subject. The performative is "that discursive practice that enacts or produces that which it names"[59] but whenever the speech becomes an act, the declaration depends not only on the declarant: when the mayor or the judge pronounce their phrase, they accomplish an act wherein the realization depends on a long series of repetitions, codes, contexts, rituals and recitations or re-citations which extensively surpass the moment of speech. To marry, to place a bet, to promise, are more than simple declarations and are veritable acts that, if the adequate conditions are not met, risk failure.[60] Declaring a gender identity, a sexual orientation, in saying that one is man or woman, or declaring oneself lesbian or homosexual, trans or *queer*... can all be read as examples of such linguistic procedures that fall within this register.

For Butler, the medical declaration, before birth even of "it's a boy" or "it's a girl" produces what is named. From this moment of nomination, the movement which materializes the gender of the body is set into motion, with all of the attendant expectations, injunctions, limitations, warnings, etc. Gender as a performative act amounts to affirming that, from birth, we play at femininity and masculinity on a daily basis. We play out this performance and are made to play it out. This is, without a doubt not so very different from the famous Lacanian adage "there's no such thing as Woman."[61] Effectively, from Butler's point of view, true women do not exist. They remain a sort of unattainable ideal. That said, for the philosopher, *man* does not exist either. The recited performances of gender are systematically destined to fall short of their goal: no one truly incarnates masculinity or femininity, even though each and every one is forced to endlessly and repetitively strain themselves in this direction. "That the gendered body is performative suggests that it has no ontological status apart from the various acts which constitute its reality."[62] We are constrained and forced to repeat these gestures, these formulae, these attitudes, this suffering and these postures which are attached to a masculine or feminine identity. Nevertheless, in insisting on the performative characteristic of gender, we can also gain a capacity for action.

> That gender reality is created through sustained social performances means that the very notions of an essential sex and a true or abiding masculinity or femininity are also constituted as part of the strategy that conceals gender's performative character and the performative possibilities for proliferating gender configurations outside the restricting frames of masculinist domination and compulsory heterosexuality.[63]

At bottom, we are faced with a theatre where the more false it is, the truer it rings.[64] If our identities are normed, and not naturally inherited, if they are iterative and thus subject to dissemination, rupture, modification, and repetitive transformation, then inequality, inherent in masculine domination and heterosexism, does not amount to an unshakable symbolic violence, nor a propensity that is, to such a degree, immutably inscribed within each and every one of us. Identity is never anything other than a counterfeit, a parody that can be differently played out. The figure of the *drag queen* in a distortion of the *femme fatale* allows us to understand that women themselves are shown to be "a copy, and an inevitably failed one, an ideal that no one can embody. In this sense, laughter emerges in the realization that all along the original was derived."[65] This peal of laughter resounds at length. It is communicative. It lays siege to numerous strongholds of thought. It unites new communities. As Butler underlines, "Hence, there is a subversive laughter in the pastiche-effect of parodic practices in which the original, the authentic, and the real are themselves constituted as effects."[66] Once the masks of femininity and virility have fallen, the remaining repartitions begin to teeter.

De-constructing gender, calling the binary structure into question, denaturalizing sexuality does not, by any means, imply the complete and utter disappearance of the categories of man, woman, or of masculine or feminine qualities, or of homosexual or heterosexual preferences. They are a means to an end. As Butler explains: "I went to many meetings, bars, and marches and saw many kinds of genders."[67] In insisting on the performative production of the masculine and the feminine, in casting off the ballast of ontological naturalism, the possibility of the production of "transgender" figures sees the light of day.

> This radical formulation of the sex/gender distinction suggests that sexed bodies can be the occasion for a number of different genders, and further, that gender itself need not be restricted to the usual two. If sex does not limit gender, then perhaps there are genders, ways of culturally interpreting the sexed body, that are in no way restricted by the apparent duality of sex.[68]

These multiplied identities are thus no longer drawn towards the pathologizing terms of psychosis, perversion, or aberration, but are simply other productions sharing equal status with the feminine or the masculine.

The limits of performance

Perceiving the construction of sexual identity by means of productive performance, midway between the linguistic and the parodic considerably lightens the moralistic heft that weighs upon the sexual order. Different to the theatre and its codifications – regarding text, stage direction and mechanics – this performance can occur everywhere: it is drawn up, carried out, and imposed, calling into question the established codes so as to freely occupy space. Matters and gestures are no longer directed or oriented by the transcendence of an Author or of a Text but may vary with ever more unpredictability.

However, by inscribing gender upon the performative stage, and not within the performance itself, Butler escapes the trap of a pure and simple alienation such as can be understood within the society of the spectacle. True, gender is constructed and performed. But it would lose its liberatory momentum if it was reduced to a mere effect of outrageous liberalism or enmeshed in the ideals of the *American dream*, where each and every one presented themselves as a *self-made-man, self-made-woman*, or even *self-made-whatever*... If this was the case, gender would only be limited to an egotistic capitalist whim, an artifice of advertising rhetoric. As we have illustrated through the work of J.L. Austin, above, it is not merely necessary to say the words, but to say them within the appropriate circumstances such that a performative speech act may take place.[69] Such a remark applies the brakes on any relativist vindication regarding sexuality. Rather, it invites us to draw up the genealogical chart of the manner in which we constitute ourselves.

One thus clears away the right to a limited and private jouissance, to the recognition of possible particularities, and to a consumerist vindication of narcissism. Thus envisaged, gender is constitutive of a hybrid and fertile terrain which does not stand for the particularly neoliberal relativist *doxa* where "everyone does as he pleases, as long as it is profitable," but rather represents a critical tool which is capable of considering other manners of living together.

The efficacity of Butler's discourse is two-fold. On one hand the repetition of the call to conform to norms in a performative manner wounds us, is injurious, and stigmatizes those who cannot thus identify themselves.[70] Because language marks the body, it can victimize us, hurt us. But this effect can also be reversed: leading to surprise. Minorities can therein find alternative discourses, re-signifying their existing speech to better be heard. And, as violently as they had been stigmatized by a disqualifying discourse, they would be able to forcefully sound out their capacity to modify norms reified as established facts, self-evident, and natural essences.

In fact, the prerequisite condition for the success of the performative lies in not being the mere appendage of a meagre solipsism. In order to be fulfilled, it refers to the necessary existence, not so much of a communitarianism, but of an us, an intentional community, a being together. Understood in this manner, the performative slogan does not correspond to a strict identitarian demand which would suppose the affirmation of an individualistic ego, quite the contrary. Defeated by linguistic violence, we can reappropriate it and circulate it in an alternate manner. The same goes for "*queer*" as an insult, of course, which has itself been transformed into a clarion call for unity, a field of study, a banner. Leaving the individualist paradigm behind opens up a space for movements that are constitutive, affiliative, plural, in short subjectivations which are far more open and vast than any unequivocal and closed definitional determination. It avoids any closure fixed upon an imaginary identification with the same. The *queer* uptake of the performative is not a case of simply being together, of starting out from the same point in order to stand together, but rather represents a becoming together in order to affirm difference.

Gender Trouble provoked a polemic. Accused of having forgotten the body, it was also accused of having made use of simple linguistic determinations which scorned concrete, corporeal, psychological materiality. Butler addresses and clarifies this in *Bodies That Matter, On the Discursive Limits of "Sex."* [71] Her foundational work remains nonetheless a source of reformulation and of subversive inspiration, rendering impossible the spontaneous apprehension of humanity as constituted of two, and only two, genders which would be complementary. Her invitation to reappropriate hateful discourses allows them to be deflected and allows for their reach and violence to be interrogated, questioning their whys and wherefores up until the point where they can be made fun of, in both senses of the term. They are, no longer, a cause of suffering, or require indifference. The foolishness of their foundational lack is laid bare. Collective identities which have hitherto been held to silence, have cultivated this fertile terrain composed of self-affirmation and which would not have seen the light of day if they had remained solitary, private, and idiosyncratic.

Butler does not limit herself to thumbing her nose at gender in the manner of a canonical anthropologist. Her infectious laugh seizes hold of the psychoanalytic fortress. In fact, consider the manner in which certain psychoanalytic positions have, repeatedly, contributed to the condemnation of homosexual, trans, etc. practices, in accusing them of perversion or psychoses, in refusing them the same degree of dignity that is offered to even the most symptomatic examples of those attached to the heterosexual domain, it is evident that these discourses can also amount to hate speech. A struggle to no longer have to endure this type of peremptory affirmation has been, and continues to be, undertaken. There is not much cause for joy in this. But reading Butler leads us beyond this type of demand. She re-signifies the underlying heteronormativity, unsaid, unthought, of the psychoanalytic discourse "only because sexuality is presumed to be heterosexual, and the observer, [is] here constructed as the heterosexual male"[72] She goes so far as to question the use that is made of the subject's speech and that of the analyst such as it is laid out from the position of the analytic couch. When what is said is of a more intimate order, the conditions of enunciation go over the heads of the subjects present. This is incidentally, without a doubt, that which allows the act of speaking to induce an effect upon the real. Interpretation, the analytic act, the interruption of the psychoanalytic session are all, in truth, indicative of a before and after in the subjective trajectory of the analysand.[73] Do such linguistic gestures also, in and of themselves, participate in the performative? Does saying not also become doing in the framework of an analysis?[74] In any case, thanks to minoritarian *agency* and the performativity of gender, Butler is able to study psychoanalytic discourse not only to criticize it when it is explicitly stigmatizing but also to shift the logic by which the psyche is apprehended, to rethink the manner in which knowledge drawn from the unconscious is structured. By this the cure finds itself relieved of any and all heteronormative pitfalls. It thus forms, for all minorities, a privileged space of resistance against heterosexism.

The melancholy of gender

Let us now take a look at how the reassessment of the ontological stability of gender (being either a man *or* a woman) participates in the subversion of the phallogocentric and homocentric presuppositions of psychoanalysis. In affirming that gender is a variable social construction, Butler dislodges the observer from the observable and self-evident heterosexual facts which "generat[e] a description of sexuality in terms that promote cultural stasis as its result."[75] Alternative frameworks for understanding psychic life without the need for a matrix that takes the complementarity of male and female as its starting point can see the light of day. In this sense, among the points developed by Butler in *Gender Trouble* and pursued in her later works, one must consider the notion, or rather the demonstration of the "melancholy of gender." In Butler's prose, melancholy, malady of sadness and mourning, is overturned, becoming a powerfully sarcastic remedy for every *straight* preconception.

Thus, the concept of melancholy can no longer truly be considered as a diagnostic category, but rather as a critical element capable of analyzing the production of intelligible identities and the processes by which they are formulated. The term "melancholy" is therefore no longer used in a clinical sense, but in a cultural one. Gender and melancholy are in cahoots. Their enunciation turns out to be explosive. Here again, the philosopher shifts the concept of the psychoanalytic clinic towards a cultural analysis so as to obstruct the heterosexism, the establishment of which psychoanalysis, despite its commendable intentions, sometimes contributes to.

Freud masterfully associated mourning and melancholy. In Freudian melancholy, the object of love is lost due to separation, death, or a break in the affective bond.

> Mourning is regularly the reaction to the loss of a loved person, or to the loss of some abstraction which has taken the place of one, such as one's country, liberty, an ideal, and so on. In some people the same influences produce melancholia instead of mourning and we consequently suspect them of a pathological disposition.[76]

Freud clarifies:

> The distinguishing mental features of melancholia are a profoundly painful dejection, cessation of interest in the outside world, loss of the capacity to love, inhibition of all activity, and a lowering of the self-regarding feelings to a degree that finds utterance in self-reproaches and self-revilings and culminates in a delusional expectation of punishment.[77]

Butler takes up this logic but in order to apply it to gender. One becomes man *or* woman in mourning a prohibited and interiorized object. According to her, what we are dealing with is a form of address without addressee. She also employs the image of an "open wound" and her demonstration foments turmoil concerning the two principal cogs of "normative heterosexuality."

The latter expression is recurrent in her writing. She does not however mean that psychoanalysis would force or constrain its patients to a sort of heterosexuality. Rather, she underlines the manner in which the majority of concepts have, as their point of departure and their point of arrival, a reference to heterosexuality,[78] without this having ever been thematized in an explicit manner. By means of cultural melancholy, Butler subverts nothing less than the incest taboo and psychological bisexuality.

To be quite plain, the issue is that the Oedipal law and the interdiction against incest is preceded by a taboo that is even more fundamental: that against homosexuality. In this way, the philosopher makes an absolute mockery of the history of *straight* psychoanalysis. Her irreverence is an important milestone for a clinic in a minor key. Homosexuality no longer appears as an error in psychic development, a point at which development has been arrested, or a fixation with the completion to which heterosexuality corresponds, but represents, on the contrary, a point of departure for the operation of the psychic apparatus itself. Homosexuality no longer corresponds to an anomaly which precludes the attainments of "normal sexual life,"[79] corresponding rather to its conditions of possibility. From a logical and clinical point of view, the foreclosing of homosexuality, its prohibition, far precedes that of the Oedipal.

> the primary homosexual attachment is culturally enforced by a prohibition on homosexuality which is in no way paralleled in the case of the melancholic homosexual. In other words, heterosexual melancholy is culturally instituted and maintained as the price of stable gender identities related through oppositional desires.[80]

This strategy allows Butler to reveal the fundamental fragility of the heterosexual order. She disturbs its tendency to fail to see the manner in which it construes itself as the be all and end all of reflection. Veritably a colossus with feet of clay, the latter requires its perpetual performative repetition so as to prove its naturality and self-evident necessity (to itself). The true feat of Butler's approach is to show the degree to which this epistemological and political preconception is, in reality, little more than a psychological house of cards. The predominantly heterosexual society in which we live, the positions of sexual maturity, as defined by the Freudian orthodoxy, and even more broadly, the establishment of culture would only be possible from the starting point of a foundational taboo which was *embodied* in a melancholic manner. The fundamental interdiction, unavoidable universal, that which establishes our civilizational order, would not be, as structuralism considered by Lacan and Lévi-Strauss would have, the incest taboo, but, first and foremost, that against homosexuality. "Gender identification is a kind of melancholia in which the sex of the prohibited object is internalized as a prohibition. This prohibition sanctions and regulates discrete gendered identity and the law of heterosexual desire."[81]

On the *straight* side of things, heterosexuals do not know and do not experience homosexual love. At most, it has been sublimated.[82] Incidentally, as we recall, the Oedipus complex of the young boy orientates desire, spontaneously, towards the parent of the opposite sex. Herein, Butler's work is interested in the unconscious of the Freudian text itself. In fact, "with the postulation of a bisexual set of libidinal dispositions, there is no reason to deny an original sexual love of the son for the father, and yet Freud implicitly does."[83] When one takes this implicit aspect into account, the entire psychoanalytic structure begins to teeter.

On the *queer* side of things, we could just as well affirm that which allows for this polarization of desire towards *the* opposite sex, that which permits stable gender assignation, is only possible on account of a more profound taboo: that which forecloses the very possibility of experiencing homosexual desire.

> In other words, the object is not only lost, but the desire fully denied, such that "I never lost that person and I never loved that person, indeed never felt that kind of love at all." The melancholic preservation of that love is all the more securely safeguarded through the totalizing trajectory of the denial.[84]

The rejection of homosexuality is thus transformed into melancholic domination of homosexuality as an impossible starting point for discourse, desire, and homosexual identity. Homosexual investment is thus "subordinated to a culturally sanctioned heterosexuality."[85] Through the melancholy of gender, Butler succeeds in upending this cultural sanction. She deploys tactical mockery, together with dialectic and parodic reversal: the majority is dependent on that which it oppresses, that which it refutes, or, at best, that which it tolerates. But there is more. In making use of melancholy, in terms of a malady of impossible mourning, Butler is able to explain anew the manner in which the death drive inhabits, and exceeds, each and every subject.[86] She rekindles the fire of the impossible from whence she draws her tireless strength, beyond any dependence on anything *straight*. At the heart of the minoritarian, ex-sists an affinity with the unyielding darkness that melts away the completeness of the pleasure principle. *Beyond the Pleasure Principle* is thus inscribed beyond heteronormativity.[87]

Conjuring psychological bisexuality

Of course, we could object to Butler in stating that the homosexual component was far from absent from Freud's understanding of the libido. Repressed homosexual tendences are, incidentally, explained by psychological bisexuality.[88] It is this second cog in the machine of normative heterosexuality that Butler hastens to dismiss. She remarks that:

> the binary restriction on sexuality shows clearly that culture in no way postdates the bisexuality that it purports to repress: It constitutes the matrix of intelligibility through which primary bisexuality itself becomes thinkable. The "bisexuality" that is posited as a psychic foundation and is said to be repressed at a later date is a discursive production that claims to be prior to all discourse, effected through the compulsory and generative exclusionary practices of normative heterosexuality.[89]

Here, Butler's logic is identical to that which she employs earlier in order to invert the primacy of sex over gender. Cultural norms impose the belief in the primacy of bisexuality. In other words, Freudian bisexuality only imposes itself within the framework of truly heterosexist thought. Such bisexuality seems to have been formulated, primarily, by and for heterosexuals.

Even though Freudian psychological bisexuality can be counted among the numerous discoveries which have incited the most outrage, according to Butler, this notion only corresponds to a preconception which is necessary in order to shore up the deadlock in which *straight* reasoning finds itself. In fact, taking a closer look at the foundational texts of psychoanalysis, it is apparent that psychological bisexuality is considered in heterosexist or heteronormative terms. In his famous article "'A Child is Being Beaten' A Contribution to the Study of the Origin of Sexual Perversions" Freud writes "in the last resort we can only see that both in male and female individuals masculine as well as feminine instinctual impulses are found, and that each can equally well undergo repression and so become unconscious."[90] But this bisexuality is understood as both masculine and feminine in both the man and the woman on the condition that the subject be heterosexually orientated. Should the man have a feminine aspect within him, that feminine aspect would only desire men.[91] It would thus be able to explain masculine homosexuality.[92] The same goes for women, it is their masculine aspect which would be attracted to women. "The conceptualization of bisexuality in terms of dispositions, feminine and masculine, which have heterosexual aims as their intentional correlates, suggests that for Freud bisexuality is the coincidence of two heterosexual desires within a single psyche."[93]

What is at work, either in the promotion of bisexuality, or in advancing the incest taboo, as guarantor of humanity, is the taboo against homosexuality. I can only become a "true" woman or a "true" man in becoming, myself, the lost object of love. In the classical conception of the Oedipus complex, as in Freudian bisexuality, there is a denial of the love of each subject for their own sex. The psychoanalytic matrix will remain heteronormative for as long as it refuses to disrupt these fundamental levers of psychological construction. From the point of view of this melancholic excess, Butler explains the panicked fear that takes hold of some of us when faced with unconventional sexual behaviour or disconcerting identities. Bizarre, *queer* behaviour forces us to face the denial and mourning that the Oedipalizing structure would not have allowed us to discern. "Within Freud's thesis of primary bisexuality, there is no homosexuality, and only opposites attract."[94] Freud forgot to conjure psychological bisexuality in all its forms. The homosexual unthought thus evolves into an unthinkable and indispensable imperative. "The taboo against homosexuality in effect creates the heterosexual 'dispositions' by which the Oedipal conflict becomes possible."[95] Within the Oedipus complex, the melancholy of culture can be found: a necessary loss which allows heterosexuality to be structured as the foundation of the normality of desire.

Despair, laugh: psychoanalyse

In having so long insisted upon the heteronormative unthought of psychoanalytic metapsychology, have the principal stakes not been forgotten? What use are all of these dialectic upheavals which disturb the structures which have hitherto allowed for unconscious discourse to be understood? In too closely following the sophisticated ideas of Butler, does one not risk somewhat wantonly imperilling the psychoanalytic structure itself? Are we not able to pass judgement on psychoanalysis as heterosexist and homophobic, phallocentric, and antifeminist without being able to propose little more than a well-polished rhetorical exercise?[96] In reality, through her meticulous reading, Butler gives herself over to a performative subversive exercise that is typically *queer*. In this it is decisive that this reading allows us to better understand the manner in which psychoanalysis too often embodies the posture of a discipline orientated by *straight* reference points. Butler's deconstruction enables us to see the manner in which we have ventured into the unconscious: with concepts that belong to a school of thought that, if it is not strongly conceptualized, at the very least, and despite itself, reproduces a heteronormative domination. Being able to see this allows for an understanding of the insistent critiques levelled against psychoanalysis by sexual minorities. For all that, it is not a question of abandoning the practice, to refuse to take on analyses in so far as we lack a sufficiently "safe," "friendly," or "inclusive" analytical apparatus. Through her wily and complex reasoning, Butler incites us to cut out the unthought from our discourse concerning the psychological, the family, the sexual. In order to revitalize work on the unconscious it is only necessary to seize upon the colours of the spectrum that shine out from the margins. In following such a brightly coloured rainbow one offsets oneself twice fold.

On one hand, in the play of the deconstruction of the Oedipal and the abandonment of heterosexist preconceptions, we lose the original. It is as if Butler announced that the Oedipal, the Phallus, Man, Woman, Structure, or Heterosexuality no longer corresponded by any measure to the origins or the ends of what would be an unchanging line of thought. Psychoanalysis itself, replete with these interpretations, no longer offers an overarching view capable of having the last word regarding who and what we are. On the stage of the grand theatre of gender there is a proliferation of semblances. Perhaps Butler's use of melancholy has no direct clinical utility. It is difficult to see how a practician would make use of it when faced with someone who is truly experiencing a pathological state of mourning. The analytical references appear to be a series of precarious fictions that delude themselves into believing that they possess sovereign power. In other words, Butler reminds us, in a minor key, of that which Lacan has already explained in "The Direction of the Treatment and its Principles of Power": "An ethics must be formulated that integrates Freud's conquests concerning desire: one that would place at the forefront the question of the analyst's desire."[97]

On the other hand, leaving the *straight* referential framework invites an understanding of what is at play in the cure, not only for LGBTQIA+ minorities, but also for all the others, like so many pathways through which desire can be experienced. There is still much to do in order to realize the work of this clinic which no longer has to dovetail with any binary ideal or with the complementarity of the sexes. Nothing has changed, but nothing remains the same: the discourse of a cure consists of allowing that which the subject can formulate regarding his being to spring forth, of taking responsibility for the sites of his psychological sufferance, of circumscribing his jouissance, and of allowing his desire to emerge. But the terms and the conceptual arrangements through which these movements travel are no longer given over to the edification of meaning which is dependent on a heteronormative matrix. "Normative heterosexuality" thus sees itself stripped of its political, theoretical, moral, and clinical privileges. Butler's philosophical sleight of hand has the benefit of recalling the degree to which attentiveness to the unconscious has both ethical and political repercussions. Going without these theoretical demonstrations amounts to missing the boat regarding both our identitarian construction and as concerns the manner in which the analytic act, itself, can be seen as being in touch, or out of touch, with a series of norms that influence psychoanalytic theory itself.

Reading *Gender Trouble* irritates clinicians of both sexes. Upon each page, they bear witness to the exposition of certain principles which they have sought to hang on to in the course of the cure. Upset at having, for so long, believed in the self-evident preconceptions of their masters, they find themselves vulnerable to jeering deconstructions. But this "is not cause for despair or, at least, it is not *only* cause for despair."[98] It is true that *queer* irony threatens analytic theory. But it also brings some joy back to the *praxis*. In inverting heterosexism, we gain access to a clinical and critical manner of thinking that is capable of being at ease with a multitude of encounters on a case-by-case basis: almost as "many kinds of genders"[99] as there are people. The analytic encounter can now occur and be subsumed in a logic that is beyond the heterosexual epicentre. With every new case, new capacities for action see the light of day. Granting conceptual ease – while certainly paradoxical, but nevertheless affirmative and open – to the clinic in a minor key thus constitutes a primary approach to Butler's work. To carry this to its ultimate logical conclusion is to dare to question oneself regarding the necessity of the reference to *the* difference between the sexes in the investigation of the unconscious. We have not yet finished having a good laugh!

Notes

1 "Se nommer en tant que lesbienne (ou gay), est un pari, c'est prendre le risque qu'à tout moment la reconnaissance de l'orientation sexuelle accapare tout le sens et définisse ainsi entièrement l'individu, alors que ce n'est qu'une partie de la vie, mais qu'elle ne déterine pas pour autant toute la vie d'une personne." Natacha Chetcuti, *Se dire lesbienne* (Payot & Rivage, 2013), 135.

2 "Faites ce que vous voulez, mais de la discretion, que diable!" Natacha Chetcuti, *Se dire lesbienne*, 129.

3 This neologism superposes "history" and "hysteria" in order to allow the "mendacious truth" to be heard, which is presented when he (or she) decides to share the fruits of their own analytic experience once they deem the analysis to have been completed. Lacan referred to this procedure as "the pass." Hystory thus evokes the possibility of putting words to a subjective journey without falling into the absolutization of any belief in Truth. "All I can do is tell the truth. No, that isn't so – I have missed it. There is no truth that, in passing through awareness, does not lie" Jacques Lacan, *The Four Fundamental Concepts of Psychoanalysis. The Seminar of Jacques Lacan. Book XI 1963–1964*, ed. Jacques-Alain Miller, trans. Alan Sheridan (W.W. Norton & Company, 1978), vi. The "y" in "hystory" does not refer to the masculine biological marker of the y chromosome but rather to the never-ending short story, to the hysteric, and to Oedipus.

4 Jacques Lacan, "L'étourdit" *The Letter* 41. Translated by C. Gallagher (2009), 32. Thus Lacan moves our attention from the contents of what is said towards the fact itself that we are inhabited by language, the said.

5 "[…] c'est-à-dire le dispositive par lequel les individus se conçoivent à partir d'une norme sexuelle majoritaire, ou du moins posée comme telle, par rapport à laquelle

l'homosexualité se singularise tout en s'isolant." Natacha Chetcuti, *Se dire lesbienne*, 115.

6 Monique Wittig, "The Straight Mind" in *The Straight Mind and Other Essays* (Beacon Press, 1992), 27.

7 In French, a preliminary perspective regarding the identitarian detonation associated with queer can be read in Pierre Zoberman (ed.), *Queer: écritures de la différance?* (L'Harmattan, 2004). This subject has been covered by a vast number of publications by American authors, among which we could cite Judith Jack Halberstam, *The Queer Art of Failure* (Duke University Press, 2011) and the work of Lee Edelman, see Lee Edelman, *Homographesis: Essays in Gay Literary and Cultural Theory* (Routledge, 1994), as well as Lee Edelman, *No Future: Queer Theory and the Death Drive* (Duke University Press, 2004), Lee Edelman, "Piss Elegant: Freud, Hitchcock, and the Micturating Penis." *GLQ 1* (April 1995, 2): 149–177. doi: doi:10.1215/10642684-2-1_and_2-149 and Lee Edelman, "Against Survival: Queerness in a Time That's Out of Joint," *Shakespeare Quarterly* 62, 2 (2011): 148–69. http://www.jstor.org/stable/23025624.

8 "Invisibilisation de l'homophobie." To quote the expression coined by Claude Rabant, "La difference sexuelle n'existe pas," in *Homosexualités et stigmatisation*, ed. by Susann Heenan-Wolff (Presses Universitaires de France, 2010), 17.

9 "Poussant les choses jusqu'au bout, on devrait faire entrer l'hétérosexualité elle-même dans cette grande maison commune de la perversion." Claude Rabant, "La difference sexuelle n'existe pas," 29.

10 See Lee Edelman, *No Future: Queer Theory and the Death Drive.*

11 Gayle Rubin, "Thinking Sex: Notes for a Radical Theory of the Politics of Sexuality" in *Pleasure and Danger: Exploring Female Sexuality*, ed. by Carole S. Vance (Routledge, 1984), 279.

12 Gayle Rubin, "Thinking Sex: Notes for a Radical Theory of the Politics of Sexuality," 283.

13 Gayle Rubin, "Thinking Sex: Notes for a Radical Theory of the Politics of Sexuality," 283.

14 "[…] après tout, le sexisme n'empêche pas d'aimer les femmes. De la même manière, l'affection pour les homosexuels ne conduit pas toujours, en France aujourd'hui, à revendiquer l'égalité des sexualités…" Eric Fassin, "Le 'outing' de l'homophobie est-il de bonne politique?" in *L'Inversion de la question homosexuelle* (Editions Amsterdam, 2008), 77.

15 Lee Edelman, "The Future is Kid Stuff" in *No Future: Queer Theory and the Death Drive*, 2.

16 Sigmund Freud, "Three Essays on the Theory of Sexuality" in *The Standard Edition of the Complete Psychological Works of Sigmund Freud.* Vol. VII. Edited by James Strachey, Anna Freud, and Angela Richards. (Hogarth Press, 1953 - 1974), 191.

17 See Jonathan Ned Katz, *The Invention of Heterosexuality* (Dutton, 1995) and Thomas Laqueur, *Making Sex. Body and Gender from the Greeks to Freud* (Harvard University Press, 1990).

18 Jonathan Ned Katz, *The Invention of Heterosexuality*, 13.

19 Jonathan Ned Katz, *The Invention of Heterosexuality*, 15. Regarding this point, Katz takes advantage of the historical perspective offered by Michel Foucault, *The History of Sexuality. Volume I: An Introduction*, trans. Robert Hurley (Pantheon Books, 1978) as well as of that presented by Eve Kosofsky Sedgwick, *Epistemology of the Closet* (University of California Press, 1990).

20 Jonathan Ned Katz, *The Invention of Heterosexuality*, 57.

21 Jonathan Ned Katz, *The Invention of Heterosexuality*, 81.

22 Judith Butler, *The Psychic Life of Power, Theories in Subjection* (Stanford University Press, 1997), 138.
23 See Félix Guattari and Suely Rolnik, *Molecular Revolution in Brazil* (Semiotext(e), 2007).
24 Judith Butler, *Gender Trouble: Feminism and the Subversion of Identity* (Routledge, 1999), vii.
25 Judith Butler, *Gender Trouble*, vii.
26 Considerations in this vein, of an understanding of "normal" starting from the pathological and a consequent relativization of the strict distinction between the two are innumerable in the works of Freud. See, for instance, Sigmund Freud, "Introductory Lectures on Psychoanalysis" in *The Standard Edition of the Complete Psychological Works of Sigmund Freud*. Vol. XV. Edited by James Strachey, Anna Freud, and Angela Richards. (Hogarth Press, 1953 - 1974), 392, 404, 412–413, 433.
27 Sigmund Freud, "Three Essays on the Theory of Sexuality" in *The Standard Edition of the Complete Psychological Works of Sigmund Freud*. Vol. VII, 162.
28 Sigmund Freud, "Fragment of an Analysis of a case of Hysteria" in *The Standard Edition of the Complete Psychological Works of Sigmund Freud*. Vol. VII, 50.
29 Judith Butler, *Gender Trouble*, 43–44.
30 Judith Butler, *Gender Trouble*, 11.
31 For a transdisciplinary and historical review of the concept see Laurie Laufer and Florence Rochefort, *Qu'est-ce que le genre?* (Payot, 2014).
32 Judith Butler, *Gender Trouble*, 11.
33 Regarding this point, see the deconstruction of the natural by Christine Delphy, *L'Ennemi principal 2. Penser le genre* (Syllepse, 2009), 228: "To summarise our work in a very schematic manner, we think that gender – the respective social positions of men and women – is not constructed upon the (apparently) natural category of sex; but that, on the contrary, sex has become a pertinent fact, and thus a category of perception beginning with the creation of the category of gender, that is to say, the division of humanity into two antagonist groups where one oppresses the other, men and women." / "pour résumer de façon très schématique notre travail, nous pensons que le genre – les positions sociales respectives des femmes et des gommes – n'est pas construite sur la catégorie (apparamment) naturelle du sexe; mais qu'au contraire le sexe est devenu un fait pertinent, et donc une catégorie de la perception à partir de la création de la catégorie de genre, c'est-à-dire de la division de l'humanité en deux groupes antagonistes dont l'un opprime l'autre, les hommes et les femmes."
34 To use the terms of Maurice Merleau-Ponty, *The Visible and the Invisible*, ed. Claude Lefort, trans. Alphonso Lingis (Northwestern University Press, 1968). For a brilliant reading of this text by Butler, see Judith Butler, "Sexual Ideology and Phenomenological Description," in *The Thinking Muse, Feminism and Modern French Philosophy: A Feminist Critique of Merleau-Ponty's* Phenomenology of Perception, ed. Jeffner Allen and Iris Marion Young (Indiana University Press, 1989), 85–100.
35 Judith Butler, *Gender Trouble*, vii.
36 Judith Butler, "An Interview with Judith Butler," *The Believer*, May 1, 2003, https://www.thebeliever.net/an-interview-with-judith-butler/
37 "Chaque fois que nous essayons de faire référence au corps, nous effectuons cette référence sous certains modes de description ou selon certains cadres de référence, mais, à chaque fois, nous échouons à nous y référer: il y a quelque chose qui excède l'acte de cette référence et qui brise, dans le langage même, l'effort de

donner une reference." Judith Butler, "Le corps en pièces" in *Sexualités, genre et mélancolie,* ed. by Monique David-Ménard (Campagne Première, 2009), 214–215.

38 Here I make reference to the expression designating the dialogue that is both "conciliatory and antagonistic [...] between Freud and Foucault" coined by Léo Bersani, "Fr-oucault and the End of Sex," in *Is the Rectum a Grave? And Other Essays* (University of Chicago Press, 2010) 133–139.

39 Judith Butler, *The Psychic Life of Power, Theories in Subjection* (Stanford University Press, 1997), 20.

40 Judith Butler, *The Psychic Life of Power,* 18. Regarding Foucault's relationship with regard to psychoanalysis, one can read a particularly interesting interview conducted by, among others, Jacques-Alain Miller in Michel Foucault, "The Confession of the Flesh," in *Knowledge/Power, Selected Interviews and Other Writings 1972–1977,* ed. by Colin Gordon, trans. by Colin Gordon, Leo Marshall, John Mepham and Kate Soper (Pantheon Books, 1980), 194–228.

41 His initial interest was transformed into hate, denouncing psychoanalysis as an exercise of power. In the end, in *The History of Sexuality,* praxis is assimilated to a discipline that aims at a confession of the truth supporting nothing other than an illusory liberty. In short, a biopower technique that aims at taming desire and spoiling pleasure. Concerning the ambiguity of the relationship that Foucault had to psychoanalysis see the excellent journal *Incidence.* "Foucault avec la psychanalyse," *Incidence* 4–5 (2009).

42 In France the work of Sam Bourcier is, without a doubt, the most advanced as regards this question. See Marie-Hélène Sam Bourcier, *Queer Zone. Politique des identités sexuelles, des representations et des savoirs* (Editions Amsterdam, 2006) as well as Marie-Hélène Sam Bourcier, *Queer Zone 2* (Editions Amsterdam, 2006) and Marie-Hélène Sam Bourcier, *Queer Zone 3* (Editions Amsterdam, 2006).

43 Regarding this point, see the critiques of *Gender Trouble* at the "antinaturalist" perspective in Stéphane Haber, *Critique de l'antinaturalisme* (Presses Universitaires de France, 2006).

44 Judith Butler, *The Psychic Life of Power,* 29.

45 This is also Léo Bersani's hypothesis, see Léo Bersani, "Fr-oucault and the End of Sex."

46 Michel Foucault, *The History of Sexuality. Volume I: An Introduction,* 91.

47 Judith Butler, *The Psychic Life of Power,* 11.

48 Judith Butler, *The Psychic Life of Power,* 14–15.

49 Judith Butler, *The Psychic Life of Power,* 17.

50 Regarding this point and for a contribution to the politics of performativity, see Judith Butler and Athena Athanasiou, *Dispossession: The Performative in the Political* (Polity, 2013) and Judith Butler, *Notes Toward a Performative Theory of Assembly* (Harvard University Press, 2015).

51 Judith Butler, *Frames of War. When is Life Grievable?* (Verso, 2009), 170.

52 Judith Butler, *Frames of War,* 170.

53 Judith Butler, *Frames of War,* 170–171.

54 Sigmund Freud, "On Beginning the Treatment (Further Recommendations on the Technique of Psycho-Analysis I)" in *The Standard Edition of the Complete Psychological Works of Sigmund Freud.* Vol. XII, 135.

55 Jacques Lacan, "The Direction of the Treatment and the Principles of Its Power," in *Ecrits,* trans. Bruce Fink (W.W. Norton & Company, 2006), 525 and 528.

56 Judith Butler, *The Psychic Life of Power,* 20.

57 Sigmund Freud, "On Psycho-analysis" in *The Standard Edition of the Complete Psychological Works of Sigmund Freud.* Vol. XII, 207.

58 For an introduction to the history of performance see RoseLee Goldberg, *Performance Art From Futurism to the Present*, 3rd Ed. (Thames & Hudson, 2011). See also Carole Boulbès (ed.), *Femmes, attitudes performatives aux lisières de la performance et de la danse* (Presses du Réel, 2012). Finally, to frame the links between fine art and considerations of gender, see the work of Fabienne Dumont, *La Rébellion du deuxième sexe. L'histoire de l'art au cribble des theories feminists anglo-américaines (1970–2000)* (Presses du Réel, 2011).
59 Judith Butler, *Bodies That Matter, On the Discursive Limits of "Sex"* (Routledge, 1993), 13.
60 See John L. Austin, *How to Do Things with Words* (Oxford University Press, 1962), 13–19.
61 Jacques Lacan, *The Seminar of Jacques Lacan. On Feminine Sexuality, The Limits of Love and Knowledge,* Book XX, ed. Jacques-Alain Miller, trans. Bruce Fink (W. W. Norton & Company, 1998), 72.
62 Judith Butler, *Gender Trouble*, 173.
63 Judith Butler, *Gender Trouble*, 180.
64 See Anne-Emmanuelle Berger, *Le Grand Théâtre du genre* (Belin, 2013), 19–72.
65 Judith Butler, *Gender Trouble*, 176.
66 Judith Butler, *Gender Trouble*, 186–187.
67 Judith Butler, *Gender Trouble*, xvi.
68 Judith Butler, *Gender Trouble*, 142–143.
69 John L. Austin, *How to Do Things with Words*, 13.
70 This is what Butler develops in Judith Butler, *Excitable Speech. A Politics of the Performative* (Routledge, 1997).
71 Judith Butler, *Bodies That Matter.*
72 Judith Butler, *Gender Trouble*, 63.
73 See the recently published seminar Jacques Lacan, *L'acte psychanalytique. Le Séminaire de Jacques Lacan. Livre XV.* Ed. Jacques-Alain Miller (Seuil, 2024). This seminar has been unofficially translated into English by Cormac Gallagher and is available online at http://www.lacaninireland.com/web/wp-content/uploads/2010/06/Book-15-The-Psychoanalytical-Act.pdf. See also his translation of Jacques Lacan, "Overview of the Psychoanalytic Act," trans. Cormac Gallagher. *The Letter* 18 (2000), 104–114.
74 This is what Sabine Prokhoris suggests in Sabine Prokhoris, *Le sexe prescrit. La différence sexuelle en question* (Aubier, 2000), 48, 71 and 107. See also Sabine Prokhoris, "The Prescribed Sex" in *Contemporary French Feminism*, ed. Kelly Oliver and Lisa Walsh (Oxford University Press, 2004): 177–200.
75 Judith Butler, *Gender Trouble*, 71.
76 Sigmund Freud, "Mourning and Melancholia" in *The Standard Edition of the Complete Psychological Works of Sigmund Freud.* Vol. XIV, 243.
77 Sigmund Freud, "Mourning and Melancholia," 244.
78 Quite an explicit example of this can be found in the infamous conference "Femininity," Sigmund Freud, "Femininity" in *The Standard Edition of the Complete Psychological Works of Sigmund Freud.* Vol. XXII, 112–135. For a salutary critique of this text see Luce Irigaray, "The Blind Spot of an Old Dream of Symmetry," in *Speculum of the Other Woman*, trans. Gillian C. Gill (Cornell University Press, 1985), 11–127. As Irigaray remarks, the articulation of feminine sexuality in Freud is heavily submissive as concerns masculine sexuality (see page 16).
79 This expression is frequently used by Freud. See Sigmund Freud, "Three Essays on the Theory of Sexuality" in *The Standard Edition of the Complete Psychological Works of Sigmund Freud.* Vol. VII, 123–246.

80 Judith Butler, *Gender Trouble*, 89.
81 Judith Butler, *Gender Trouble*, 80.
82 See, Sigmund Freud, "Group Psychology and the Analysis of the Ego" in *The Standard Edition of the Complete Psychological Works of Sigmund Freud*. Vol. XVIII, 67–145. Herein homosexual love is sublimated for the development of humanity (103), explained as a fixation and an identification with the mother in terms of "the model of what has hitherto been the object" (108–109), which neatly establishes the heteronormative logic from which Freud explains homosexuality (to himself) as well as how such homosexual love "desexualized, sublimated homosexual love for other men, [...] springs from work in common" (103) and thus allows us to better understand the operation of desexualized groups such as the church or the army.
83 Judith Butler, *Gender Trouble*, 75. To this end, the work of the Italian cineast Pier Paolo Pasolini develops an aesthetic which offers an alternative to the domination of the Oedipal myth by illustrating continual variations of the tortured love of a son for his father. Allow me to refer you to Fabrice Bourlez, *Pulsions pasoliniennes* (Les Presses du Réel, 2015).
84 Judith Butler, *Gender Trouble*, 88.
85 Judith Butler, *Gender Trouble*, 76.
86 Concerning this question, the place of "queerness" as a source of anxiety in the *straight* community and as an incarnation of the death drive in so far as it "also names the jouissance forbidden by, but permeating, the Symbolic order itself." See Lee Edelman, *No Future*, 27. For a discussion of Butler's positions concerning the real (positions that will be considered in the following chapter) see Lee Edelman, *No Future*, 102–107.
87 See Sigmund Freud, "Beyond the Pleasure Principle" in *The Standard Edition of the Complete Psychological Works of Sigmund Freud*. Vol. XVIII, 3–66.
88 Concerning bisexuality in Freud, see Sigmund Freud, "Three Essays on the Theory of Sexuality" in *The Standard Edition of the Complete Psychological Works of Sigmund Freud*. Vol. VII, 219–220 and the note in Sigmund Freud, "Civilisation and its Discontents" in *The Standard Edition of the Complete Psychological Works of Sigmund Freud*. Vol. XXI, 105–106. Also see the excellent work by Lionel Le Corre, *L'Homosexualité de Freud* (Presses Universitaires de France, 2017).
89 Judith Butler, *Gender Trouble*, 69–70.
90 Sigmund Freud, "'A Child is Being Beaten': A Contribution to the Study of the Origin of Sexual Perversions" in *The Standard Edition of the Complete Psychological Works of Sigmund Freud*. Vol. XVII, 202.
91 See Sigmund Freud, "Three Essays on the Theory of Sexuality" in *The Standard Edition of the Complete Psychological Works of Sigmund Freud*. Vol. VII, 219–220.
92 See Sigmund Freud, "Three Essays on the Theory of Sexuality" in *The Standard Edition of the Complete Psychological Works of Sigmund Freud*. Vol. VII, 144–146.
93 Judith Butler, *Gender Trouble*, 77.
94 Judith Butler, *Gender Trouble*, 78.
95 Judith Butler, *Gender Trouble*, 82.
96 This is one of the primary critiques levelled at Butler by Marta Nussbaum, "The Professor of Parody: The hip defeatism of Judith Butler," *The New Republic*, February 22, 1999. https://newrepublic.com/article/150687/professor-parody
97 Jacques Lacan, "The Direction of the Treatment and the Principles of Its Power," in *Ecrits*, 514.

98 Judith Butler, *Gender Trouble*, 181.
99 Judith Butler, *Gender Trouble*, xvi.

Bibliography

Austin, John L. *How to Do Things with Words*. Oxford University Press, 1962.

Berger, Anne-Emmanuelle. *Le Grand Théâtre du genre*. Belin, 2013.

Bersani, Léo. "Fr-oucault and the End of Sex." In *Is the Rectum a Grave? And Other Essays*. University of Chicago Press, 2010, 133–139.

Boulbès, Carole (ed.). *Femmes, attitudes performatives aux lisières de la performance et de la danse*. Presses du Réel, 2012.

Bourcier, Marie-Hélène Sam. *Queer Zone. Politique des identités sexuelles, des representations et des savoirs*. Editions Amsterdam, 2006.

Bourcier, Marie-Hélène Sam. *Queer Zone 2*. Editions Amsterdam, 2006.

Bourcier, Marie-Hélène Sam. *Queer Zone 3*. Editions Amsterdam, 2006.

Bourlez, Fabrice. *Pulsions pasoliniennes*. Les Presses du Réel, 2015.

Butler, Judith. "Sexual Ideology and Phenomenological Description: A Feminist Critique of Merleau-Ponty's *Phenomenology of Perception*." In *The Thinking Muse, Feminism and Modern French Philosophy*. Edited by Jeffner Allen and Iris Marion Young. Indiana University Press, 1989, 85–100.

Butler, Judith. *Bodies That Matter, On the Discursive Limits of "Sex"*. Routledge, 1993.

Butler, Judith. *Excitable Speech. A Politics of the Performative*. Routledge, 1997.

Butler, Judith. *The Psychic Life of Power, Theories in Subjection*. Stanford University Press, 1997.

Butler, Judith. Gender Trouble: Feminism and the Subversion of Identity. Routledge, 1999.

Butler, Judith. "An Interview with Judith Butler." *The Believer*. May 1, 2003. https://www.thebeliever.net/an-interview-with-judith-butler/.

Butler, Judith. *Frames of War. When is Life Grievable?*Verso, 2009.

Butler, Judith. "Le corps en pièces." In *Sexualités, genre et mélancolie*. Edited by Monique David-Ménard. Campagne Première, 2009, 214–215.

Butler, Judith. *Notes Toward a Performative Theory of Assembly*. Harvard University Press, 2015.

Butler, Judith and Athena Athanasiou. *Dispossession: The Performative in the Political*. Polity, 2013.

Chetcuti, Natacha. *Se dire lesbienne*. Payot & Rivage, 2013.

Delphy, Christine. *L'Ennemi principal 2. Penser le genre*. Syllepse, 2009.

Dumont, Fabienne. *La Rébellion du deuxième sexe. L'histoire de l'art au cribble des theories feminists anglo-américaines (1970–2000)*. Presses du Réel, 2011.

Edelman, Lee. *Homographesis: Essays in Gay Literary and Cultural Theory*. Routledge, 1994.

Edelman, Lee. "Piss Elegant: Freud, Hitchcock, and the Micturating Penis." *GLQ* 1, 2 (April 1995): 149–177. doi:10.1215/10642684-2-1_and_2-149.

Edelman, Lee. *No Future: Queer Theory and the Death Drive*. Duke University Press, 2004.

Edelman, Lee. "Against Survival: Queerness in a Time That's Out of Joint." *Shakespeare Quarterly* 62, 2 (2011): 148–169. http://www.jstor.org/stable/23025624.

Fassin, Eric. *L'Inversion de la question homosexuelle.* Editions Amsterdam, 2008.

Foucault, Michel. *The History of Sexuality. Volume I: An Introduction.* Translated by Robert Hurley. Pantheon Books, 1978.

Foucault, Michel. "The Confession of the Flesh." In *Knowledge/Power, Selected Interviews and Other Writings 1972–1977.* Edited by Colin Gordon. Translated by Colin Gordon, Leo Marshall, John Mepham and Kate Soper. Pantheon Books, 1980, 194–228.

Freud, Sigmund. *The Standard Edition of the Complete Psychological Works of Sigmund Freud.* Edited by James Strachey, Anna Freud, and Angela Richards. Hogarth Press, 1953–1974.

Goldberg, RoseLee. *Performance Art From Futurism to the Present*, 3rd Ed. Thames & Hudson, 2011.

Guattari, Félix and Suely Rolnik. *Molecular Revolution in Brazil.* Semiotext(e), 2007.

Haber, Stéphane. *Critique de l'antinaturalisme.* Presses Universitaires de France, 2006.

Halberstam, Judith Jack. *The Queer Art of Failure.* Duke University Press, 2011.

Incidence. "Foucault avec la psychanalyse," *Incidence* 4–5 (2009).

Irigaray, Luce. *Speculum of the Other Woman.* Translated by Gillian C. Gill. Cornell University Press, 1985.

Katz, Jonathan Ned. *The Invention of Heterosexuality.* Dutton, 1995.

Lacan, Jacques. *The Four Fundamental Concepts of Psychoanalysis. The Seminar of Jacques Lacan. Book XI 1963–1964.* Edited by Jacques-Alain Miller. Translated by Alan Sheridan. W.W. Norton & Company, 1978.

Lacan, Jacques. *On Feminine Sexuality, The Limits of Love and Knowledge. The Seminar of Jacques Lacan.* Book XX. Edited by Jacques-Alain Miller. Translated by Bruce Fink. W.W. Norton & Company, 1998.

Lacan, Jacques. "Overview of the Psychoanalytic Act." *The Letter* 18. Translated by Cormac Gallagher. (2000), 104–114.

Lacan, Jacques. *Ecrits*, trans. Bruce Fink. W.W. Norton & Company, 2006.

Lacan, Jacques. "L'étourdit." Translated by C. Gallagher. *The Letter* 41. (2009), 31–80.

Lacan, Jacques. *L'acte psychanalytique. Le Séminaire de Jacques Lacan. Livre XV.* Edited by Jacques-Alain Miller. Seuil, 2024.

Laqueur, Thomas. *Making Sex. Body and Gender from the Greeks to Freud.* Harvard University Press, 1990.

Laufer, Laurie and Florence Rochefort. *Qu'est-ce que le genre?*Payot, 2014.

Le Corre, Lionel. *L'Homosexualité de Freud.* Presses Universitaires de France, 2017.

Merleau-Ponty, Maurice. *The Visible and the Invisible.* Edited by Claude Lefort. Translated by Alphonso Lingis. Northwestern University Press, 1968.

Nussbaum, Marta. "The Professor of Parody: The Hip Defeatism of Judith Butler," *The New Republic*, February 22, 1999. https://newrepublic.com/article/150687/professor-parody.

Prokhoris, Sabine. *Le sexe prescrit. La différence sexuelle en question.* Aubier, 2000.

Prokhoris, Sabine. "The Prescribed Sex" in *Contemporary French Feminism.* Edited by Kelly Oliver and Lisa Walsh. Oxford University Press, 2004: 177–200.

Rabant, Claude. "La difference sexuelle n'existe pas." In *Homosexualités et stigmatisation.* Edited by Susann Heenan-Wolff. Presses Universitaires de France, 2010.

Rubin, Gayle. "Thinking Sex: Notes for a Radical Theory of the Politics of Sexuality." In *Pleasure and Danger: Exploring Female Sexuality.* Edited by Carole S. Vance. Routledge, 1984, 267–319.

Sedgwick, Eve Kosofsky. *Epistemology of the Closet.* University of California Press, 1990.

Wittig, Monique. *The Straight Mind and Other Essays.* Beacon Press, 1992.

Zoberman, Pierre (ed.). *Queer: écritures de la différance?*L'Harmattan, 2004.

Chapter 5

Beyond Sexual Difference

Fabrice Bourlez

Embracing in the boxing ring?

Let us take another look at what we have seen. To lay things out in a schematic manner, on one side, we have the *queer* who, in the wake of Foucault, Deleuze, and Guattari, consider that psychoanalysis has remained centred on the phallus and the Oedipal law. On the other side we have the psychoanalysts who defend their *praxis* against an imaginary approach, one that offers a normative and social understanding of sexuality. For the *queer*, the analysts represent the guardians of the symbolic temple, heteronormative moralizers. For the analysts, the *queer* are incapable of fixing sexuality to the field of a symbolic Other.[1] As a consequence, they remain blind when faced with the real that is in play in the drive.

One could amuse oneself in giving extensive attention to this opposition between *queer* and psychoanalytic theory. Seeing them as locked in a bloody fight where a sort of impossible dialogue could be found. Setting the stage with wayward bodies which defy all norms, the bile of the *queer* would be disgorged upon the only brace of the symbolic. Thus envisaged, their little poststructuralist games and their irreverent mockeries would not seriously endanger the psychanalytic clinic. In not having taken the real into account, the fiefdom of *queer* theory would be limited to the social and the imaginary. And, in so doing, they would miss out on the most subversive of the psychoanalytic advances. The two fields would thus no longer have anything to say to each other. The theoretical contortions, while quite stimulating at first blush, have wasted no time in fading. The importance even of this struggle, as desperate and jubilatory as it has been, would arouse less enthusiasm. And the analysts would resume their work. And the *queer* would continue their fight, vociferously, against the excesses.

But, under these circumstances, on one side, as on the other, after having followed the match between the *queer* and the analysts, blow by blow, there are only losers. Too rapidly ejected from the boxing ring, there was not enough time to learn from their hand-to-hand fight. The clinic in a major key, no doubt opts for settling this conflict in such a rapid manner. It prefers

DOI: 10.4324/9781003612735-5

to ensure the stability of its past glories than to tire itself by responding to low blows. By the by, it has little to gain: at worst, this exercise can be cast as homophobic, at best, heteronormative. For the clinic in a major key, a draw is preferable to a waste of time

On the contrary, the clinic in a minor key plays on the prolongation of the bout. Aware of the work of Judith Butler, it does not hesitate to exemplify continuous variations of the metapsychological concepts of Freud, Lacan, and their disciples. By means of impure genealogies, it is able to assess the degree of oppression that minorities face. Through irony, the clinic in a minor key does not weigh itself down with a "normative heterosexuality." It permits desire in difference and across genders. Very well. This is an engagement which once again becomes an embrace. But the real, such as Lacan has theorized it, is it not that which becomes a yawning gap in the hollow of every embrace? Does it not undermine the joyfully naïve reconciliatory optimism of the minor clinic? Let us unfold this question in more detail before adjourning the match.

The real and the *objet a*

Let us recall that the real and reality are not identical for Lacan. The real is a point of impossibility which characterizes the body of the speaking being. It is that which suspends our certitudes, that which tirelessly returns to the same position despite the best of our resolutions, the strongest effort of will, or the soundest (or most unsound) of reasons that we can offer unto ourselves. The real erupts where the jouissance of the symptom manifests in its basest form. Lacan clarifies this register of analytic experience in a decisive manner when he introduces a further element to his algebra: "the *objet a.*"

In fact, in the course of his teachings, Lacan progressively approached the significance of the phallic from an angle that wound up calling the absolute nature of the symbolic into question. True, the signifiers continue to determine our being in the world, but they are also indicative of a remainder that they seem incapable of signifying. This remainder, which is "impossible to speak" was pinpointed, not through the aid of a signifier but through the use of a simple letter, a matheme: the *objet a.*

One speaks a lot in the course of a cure, one says, repeats, elaborates, works through. But, on the whole, the attempt that is made wanes and remains shallow: it is not able to drain the space where waves of words unceasingly spring forth in a chain of constructions, of fragile flights of fancy. What all of these words dwell on and seek to express is denied, to the point of exhaustion.

Repetition conceived of as real, refers back to the movement of the drive itself, which, contrary to any need, unceasingly insists beyond any means of satisfaction. "Characterized by repetition rather than by development, the drive does not necessarily work toward the subject's well-being."[2] *Beyond the*

Pleasure Principle the subject remains attached to the repetition which leads him to relive unpleasant situations again and again. This is, for example, the case of he or she who, having suffered an accident, would unceasingly continue to relive it in his or her dreams.[3] From the starting point of this non-supremacy of the principle of pleasure within psychological economics and the observation of behaviour conditioned by repetition that is as automatic as it is mortiferous, Lacan brings the *objet a* into focus. With this matheme, in opposition to his rereading of the canonical texts concerning the formation of the unconscious (*The Interpretation of Dreams, Jokes and their Relation to the Unconscious, Psychopathology of Everyday Life*) Lacan does not so much glorify the "unconscious [...] structured like a language" than a disturbing silence that compels us to relive disagreeable experiences. The real of this silent repetition does not correspond to an unchanging essence but to the *result of the action of signification upon our bodies.* Its conception depends upon our inscription within language in so far as the latter confronts us with an impossibility which cannot be sutured by the *said.* To be in language is to accept that there will always be something to be said, that discourse will never attain a finite totality. The *objet a* is precisely the remainder of this erasure that the signifier effects upon our bodies: pleasing plenitudes that are forever lost. Thus, the *objet a* appears "embodied," as an unsymbolizable remainder of the division of the image of the body by the signifier. It is what shields us from organicism, once the repercussions of the signifier upon our being have been accepted. Lacan gives four variations: the breast, the faeces, the voice, the gaze.[4] A paradoxical point of resistance, the *objet a* "reappears in the body, in any of the parts of the body where a passage between the inside and the outside would exist."[5] In short the *objet a* is "extimate," more intimate than any interior and more distant than any exterior: a truly "foreign body."[6]

The *objet a* as a corporeal remainder thus invites the psychoanalyst to leave behind the impasses that the imaginary straitjacket that anatomical laws still imposed upon him during the Freudian period. Its "extimate" position in relation to the symbolic register also allows for the possibility of the resignification of the customs regarding the body, beyond identitarian and gender definition. The *objet a* indicates a separation that is inclusive of the real within the symbolic. In other words, the possibility of approaching the real through the apparatus of the signifier exists, even if it is impossible to express. If the real refuses its expression through words, and given that it returns to the same position, it is because it is situated at the heart of sexual jouissance. With this in mind, the queer theoretician Tim Dean clarifies:

> Freud's separation of sexuality from genitality – a separation that decisively loosens the grip of heteronormativity on our thinking – was reconceived by Lacan in terms of jouissance and the objet petit a. As the cause not the aim of desire, objet a deheterosexualizes desire by revealing

> its origin in the effects of language, rather than the effects of the opposite sex. His insistence that jouissance is not reducible to sex – like Foucault's demonstration of the historically contingent relation that sex bears to identity – represents another way of pointing to the comparatively incidental place of genitalia in sexuality.
>
> Hence the Lacanian category of jouissance could be extremely useful to the kinds of analysis that interest queer theory.[7]

In the same manner, due to its removal from the body as mediated by the signifier, Javier Saez programmatically affirms that: "The fact that the *objet a* is independent of gender (it is neither masculine nor feminine) will allow for the establishment of a non heterocentrist reading of psychoanalysis."[8] The *objet a* thus interrupts the ideality of language, gender, identity, sex, or love.

A embodied

Several years after having conceptualized the *objet a*, Lacan, in Seminar XX, *On Feminine Sexuality, The Limits of Love and Knowledge*, returned to the specificity of its ethics, when the latter returns to the real of jouissance. "*Encore*" or "again," which is the French title of the seminar, is also a sexual exclamation: "make love to me again!" But the title of the seminar should also be heard in terms of its French homophone "*en-corps*" or "em-bodied." Therein lies the mark of the ties that bind language to the body and the impossibility that can therefrom be deduced for one and for all. The *objet a* objects to the sexual relation between subjects. It returns them to a structural impossibility. Impossible to symbolize, it resists being sutured by meaning. It returns each and every subject to the particularity of their jouissance in so far as it is the motor which drives the singularity of the subject's desire. In this seminar, Lacan pronounces his famous aphorism "there is no such thing as a sexual relationship." Such an affirmation does not, by any means, imply that there are no sexual relations or jouissance of the organs. Humans, like animals, fuck. Nevertheless, the *parlêtres*, our bodies because they are marked by language, because they are taken up by the *objet a*, because they are subsumed to this impossible fencing in towards ourselves, have to confront the failure of the complementarity of the sexes. This impossible interlocking constrains us to abandon the sweet dream of a relationship where the beings end up reaching each other and understanding each other in the purest of intimacies. No perfect complementarity. No sweet synthesis. The *nouage* between the symbolic, the imaginary, and the real thus returns to inscribe a void within our speaking bodies that no relationship, not even a sexual one, can compensate to completion.

To the drive, elaborated by Freud in terms of a concept, Lacan is determined to bring about a *renewal in the domain of Eros.*[9] In order to do so, and in the wake of his seminar on *The Ethics of Psychoanalysis*,[10] he once again enters into a discussion with the Aristotelian doctrine. But, this time, he is not interested in *Nicomachean Ethics* which is concerned with the search for that which is good, rather Lacan turns his attention to the logic at work in *Organon*, in particular the works which analyze the linguistic cogs in the *Analytics, Topics* and *On Interpretation*.

Of course, Lacan always rereads Aristotle with Freud. In *Seminar VII*, as in *Seminar XX*, the Aristotelian order, seeking to discover the recurrence of truth, the good, or of being, where the latter are all moved by the Freudian discovery of a body haunted by the drives, occupied by this sombre excess which refuses any ideal of mastery or reason. Any reading of *On Feminine Sexuality, The Limits of Love and Knowledge* must be accompanied by a reading of *L'étourdit*:[11] an equally challenging text, written at the same time as *Seminar XX*. Drawing on the strange spelling of its title, Lacan's text recalls the opacity of the body extended along the prism of the unconscious. Through its grammatical impossibility and its graphical and phonetic polyvocality, it opens up to a beyond common signification or conscious semantics, allowing us to catch a glimpse of what the unconscious evokes in its dimension as outside-of-sense. It is in this text, written in 1972, that we can read the phrase, laconic, to say the least, and which we have already encountered several times. "That one might be saying (*Qu'on dise*) remains forgotten behind what is said in what is heard."[12] The psychoanalytic undertaking is thus articulated in the question of *saying* and its difference to what is *said* and what is *heard* or *understood*. In his precise and rigorous reading of *L'étourdit*, Christian Fierens allows us to understand that, behind the universalist appearances of each assertation, a neatly subjective dimension always lies, from the moment when listening is less attentive to the contents than it is to the fact that something has been said. "A statement exterior to what is said is called into existence through the intermediary of understanding; a *statement* exterior to understanding is called into existence through the intermediary of that which is said."[13] Thus, *what is said* insists, above all, as the absence of conscious signification, as a rupture with regards to the Ego. Thus, what draws the attention of the analyst in the course of the cure, does not so much resemble sense as it does that which distances itself from it: "ab-sense." Incidentally, the analyst himself plays at absence – often quite concretely through his silence. The singular modality of relating to language aims at locating *that which is said*. As Lacan notes, "what is said does not go without a saying."[14] If *what is said* passes through another grammar other than the truth, a universal logic, it can never untie itself from this ab-sense saying. Further on, Lacan continues: "Freud puts us on the track of the fact that lack-of-sense (*ab-sens*) designates sex."[15]

In a simplified manner, let us say that Lacan distinguishes two forms of listening: on one hand, attention would be paid to *what is said* which makes sense (a promise of truth, universality, rich in conceptual architecture, far removed from the baseness of the flesh, in short "ab-sex". This would permit the classification of individuals following logical and rational categories. Intersubjectivity establishes itself communally on this *relationship* of signification. Here, between the imaginary and the symbolic, the perception of *reality* is tied. On the other hand, a *saying* which should be decoupled from *what is said*. This *saying* is characterized by an absence of signification in so far as it designates an "ab-sense sex." Fierens explains:

> The suspension of signification in the practice of free association reveals the subject of sex as concerns the speaker. This question does not find a satisfying answer in the chromosomic or anatomical reality. Sex as concerns the speaker is not determined by any foundation prior to language; it is the preconceived absence of determination.[16]

The modality of the subject's jouissance flows forth from the singular manner in which each subject fixes itself within language. On the stage of the unconscious, the *nouage* of the imaginary, the symbolic and the real is undertaken. If the universal of *what is said* depends on the belief in an ab-sense sex, in speech for which the contents have value in and of themselves and could lay claim to truth, *saying* is attached to an impossible real. Thus, even if we *say* words of love, explain ourselves, hesitate, tear ourselves apart, *what is said* is irrevocable: "there is no sexual relationship."[17] The subject of the unconscious, through the impact of language, articulates in *what is said* a *saying* that compensates for this fundamental absence.

We are thus witness to the passage from a structuralist clinic, centred on tracking down signification, to a clinic where "there is no sexual relationship": a clinic of jouissance where the symptoms would be equivalent to "all the diverse fixations, the diverse modalities which grant access to the jouissance that each and every one has at their disposal, whether or not they conform to the particular norms of a given era."[18] Thus conceived, the symptom is no longer indicative of any illness whatsoever. More than a mere manner of speaking, it would mark a manner of experiencing jouissance. If psychoanalysis sets itself upon the path facing the enigma of the symptom which defies logical explanation, it is in order to, at the end of the journey, reach this point which cannot be sutured and wherefrom our singularity emerges: the rift in the real which animates us. This real defies good old common sense, communicational efficacy, commercial speech, affirmative resolutions rich with happy promises, coaching, or good health. Confining the symptom to this vision of the real, allows it to be voided of both its impact and its sense. *What is said* by the subject is not so much there to make sense as it is there to confront the lack-of-sense, this kernel of the real that defies again and again, embodies the handsome constructions of reality. Too often embroiled in our striving to understand what is said, we neglect this space from which speech emerges before it takes on sense like so many attempts at sealing off an unfillable breach.

This space of *saying* is the analytic point of reference. Such a locus is as strange as it is paradoxical: it is the void which renders signifying articulation, the movement of subjective history, possible. It leads to a frenzied quest for sense, which nothing succeeds in exhausting. This point of our subjectivity refuses any written expression. The most singular aspect of each of our beings is thus lodged in that which "doesn't stop not being written" all while refusing us any completeness whatsoever.

Thus considered, the real goes as far as to defy the notion of truth. No truth or universality can assert itself when faced with the real. Only the semblances which act as bulwarks against the collapse of ideals subsist. As Lacan states, "that what the analytic discourse concerns is the subject, which, as effect of meaning, is response to the real."[19] In other words, if, due to language, there is no sexual relationship, then there is jouissance which can also be written as "j'ouïs-sens" (*I hear sense*). The subject suffers in so far as they would like to give meaning and sense to that which refuses both meaning and sense and which nevertheless demands it. Our dysfunctions, our psychological disappointments, our malaise, our dreams and our slips of the tongue, that which is fertile ground for the *talking cure*, is only of interest in so far as it represents a response to the real which is, at the very least, disconcerting. "By becoming cognisant of the real, we alleviate its weight, all while putting an end to the vain hopes generated by the mirage of truth."[20] The symptom thus ends up signifying nothing at all. Opaque resistance to sense, it admittedly insists upon the yawning gap that is its wont. But it no longer signifies anything. One makes do.

The tables of sexuation

Based upon these reflections, Lacan establishes his formulas of sexuation. Fierens, in his reading of *L'étourdit*, offers a clear summary: "from the circuit implied by the unconscious, two universals can be identified ('the two sexes') which separate the speaking beings, not two types of being, not two genders or species, but two logics or, better, two logical parties independent of biological sex."[21]

The clinic of jouissance is thus founded upon the "formulas of sexuation," which respond point for point to the logic of Aristotle's *Organon*. [22] These formulas endeavour to see themselves as being at once indifferent to biological universalism, as to traditional social binarism as conveyed by *the* sexual difference. Nevertheless, the table upon which they are distributed is divided into nothing less than two sections: that of phallic jouissance, said to be the "man portion" and that of the Other jouissance, said to be the "woman portion."[23] On the "man" portion of the table, Lacan distributes that which, within his teaching, falls under the phallic function and castration: the law, the universal, the Oedipal, and so on. On the "woman" portion he inscribes a form of jouissance that goes beyond phallic jouissance. According to

Lacan, feminine jouissance is "not wholly" in the phallic function. Once again, the invention of the quantifier of female sexuality as "not whole" clearly runs counter to Aristotelian logic. In locating a jouissance other than phallic, Lacan designates a point of jouissance that is outside the symbolic, outside the mastery of man as imposing logic upon the world. "Woman" does thus not exist; she always manages to slip away from the phallic imperialism of the definite article. Lacan goes so far as to bar ~~Woman~~. As a consequence, *the* difference between the sexes is no longer dependant on an anatomical opposition but on this asymmetry in the relationship to jouissance and to language: female jouissance does not complement male jouissance but is radically Other. It is supplementary.

The symptom thus becomes a partner to the subject:

> It is the politics of the subject against the collectivist politics of the prevailing discourse. The politics of psychoanalysis thus has a vocation to change, somewhat, the economy of jouissance as it is established between the subject, objector of universalised jouissance, and discourse, which administers the aforementioned jouissance.[24]

Psychoanalysis thus invites the subject not so much to "govern" jouissance, as to "elucidate" it, in discovering the singularity of its desire without renouncing it, even if it contradicts the norms of the established order.

Consequently, from a *queer* point of view, there are several pressing questions: does the founding axiom – the famous "there is no such thing as a sexual relationship" – allow for the opposition between men and women to be rethought not in terms of complementarity but in terms of a veritable asymmetry capable of multiplying itself across, and in terms of, non-normative sexualities? Is this table of sexuation capable of opening itself up to particularities which would not, to any extent, be correlative to *the* difference between the sexes, taken as the sole and unique point of departure (and ultimate destination) of reflection? From a post-feminist perspective, the reapparition of a duality within the quantifiers of sexuality, and the return of an undefinable alterity, with the "not whole" jouissance on the woman portion, reestablishes, deep within our unconscious, distinctions directly descended from the patriarchy and the hierarchy of sex and of gender. In other words, does the opposition, while non-complementary or non-dialectic, of one aspect reflecting phallic jouissance on the man portion, and a "supplementary" jouissance on the woman portion, not draw on gender in order to trace its radically renewed understanding of the sexual? Indeed, in skirting the statement of the obvious, is the strict binary of the table not tributary to the profoundly dualist cultural construction? Is two the only possible foundation for an ethics of psychoanalysis? Furthermore, if the real of such jouissance is inclusively separated within the symbolic, if it is the product of a remainer of the action of language upon our bodies, if additionally, the grammar of this language is always already marked by the seal of the heteronormativity that is proper to *straight* thought, and if, finally, the signifying articulation is the effect of "a primitive ontological concept that enforces in language a division of beings into sexes,"[25] then how can the real thus conceived distinguish itself from the matrix of "normative heterosexuality"? It is time to turn back to Judith Butler.

Butler and the real

In order to defend oneself against Judith Butler's deconstructions, one could argue that the real, in the sense in which we have just advanced, is that which is wholly absent from her theory. As numerous commentators have remarked,

> she still seems to be too fixated upon her opposition to the heteronormative symbolic, inspired by Lévi-Strauss, immobilising Lacan in the era of his "return to Freud" and the completeness of the symbolic, perhaps dismissing the importance of the change that his conceptualisation has undergone as he has given more and more importance to the "real."[26]

This is the key point upon which Butler's parodies have faltered.

Affirming that Butler has not taken the real into account, is to dismiss her as a philosopher who is still overly engaged with the question of meaning. It is to argue that, despite the poststructuralist complexity of her theoretical constructions, she has not succeeded in taking on board the radicality of the Lacan's later works, which, alone, are capable of vigorously facing up to this locus of speech, profoundly indifferent to the applicable norms, the manner of doing things, or even the social. Saying, forgotten in what is heard, finds no other shore than that of the analytic couch and pays no heed to performativity. Upon this terrain there is less Oedipalization, less familial narrative, less of a requirement to pass from one stage to another, less anatomy. And yet, no less difference. The real would impose itself upon each and every speaking body in ever new and novel occurrences, unique at every turn, indifferent to the laws of signification. While Butler expends great effort in making the most excluded of lives possible, while she imposes a duty upon herself to open up our narrative patterns, while she fights to mourn all deaths without distinction, while she struggles to enlarge the patterns of our lexical, cognitive, and normative categories, while she rebels against the heterosexism of Freud and Lacan, she would only scratch the surface of, or even repress, the stakes of what is afoot in a psychoanalysis: that which is impossible to say or express, and from which arises the said, the real which labours its point in the ab-sense which is characteristic of sex. Herein the path of resistance to biopolitics, in Foucault's terms, is materialized. It is this path that the most rigorous of Lacanian psychoanalysis sets out to discover: beneath commonplace discourse, underlying the modes of jouissance hawked by unbridled capitalism, lies an impregnable subjective fortress, outside-of-sense, around which the half-said authenticity of desire is articulated.[27]

Without a doubt, the real is conspicuously absent from the bedside book of *queer* theory. Not one single word regarding the *objet a* or the real of jouissance in *Gender Trouble*. We could thus argue that the demands made by the *queer* have retained only a simplistic and incomplete reading of Lacan. In Butler's first works, one only considers, critiques, manhandles, Lacan's initial works. The Lacanians, confronted by the attacks and deconstructions of the *queer* theorists, thus respond that they have thrown the real out the window: "You believe that psychoanalysis is phallic, and you claim freedom in the construction of the body and of gender? OK. But your reading of Lacan is biased and your claims imaginary!"

Nevertheless, all appearances to the contrary, in the course of her work, Butler has well and truly undertaken an in-depth discussion of the real as formulated in the final teachings of Lacan. If she did not grasp the radicality of this register in *Gender Trouble*, it is nonetheless evident that, in the course of several works written in the wake of *Gender Trouble*, she has taken this radicality into account. This discussion is, in particular, undertaken through a critical dialogue with the work of the Slovenian philosopher, Slavoj Žižek[28] who has over the last 20 years established himself as one of the principal exponents of the later Lacan on the international scene.[29] While the two authors are in agreement regarding the construction of critical and openly leftist thought which, among other inspirations, draws on psychoanalysis as a point of departure, their debates are nevertheless sometimes quite turbulent. These debates suffer from a clear lack of direct references to the Lacanian text. They nevertheless allow Butler's position as regarding the real to be made plain.

In the course of her intellectual work, Butler has not limited herself to a critical account of Lacanian psychoanalysis which would be limited to the phallus and the signifier. From *Bodies that Matter*, published in 1993 and directly following *Gender Trouble*, Butler has undertaken what can truly be described as a "heated debate with the real."

The limits of the performative

As Judith Butler herself underlines in the preface to *Bodies that Matter* "Theorizing from the ruins of the Logos invites the following question: 'What about the materiality of the body?'"[30] Is this materiality not profoundly dual, polarized from the dawn of time between masculine and feminine?[31] Does the real of two, and only two, sexes non suspend the excess of postmodern relativism so well adapted to the hedonist *doxa* and the triumph of the market economy? Are we not, despite the most adept and refined theorizations, entitled to seize hold of this materiality, this insistent excess of the body, as a formidable weapon to definitively bring the joyous pantomimes of genre to a close?[32]

When Žižek takes up his account of the Lacanian orientation so as to couple it to Marxist philosophy, he considers that poststructuralism, embodied in both fluidity and in Butler's parodical proliferations of gender, does not go far enough.

> Postmodern politics definitely has the great merit that it "repoliticizes" a series of domains previously considered "apolitical" or "private"; the fact remains, however, that it does not in fact repoliticize capitalism, because the very notion and form of the "political" within which it operates is grounded in the 'depoliticization' of the economy.[33]

In other words, the subversions of gender trouble are nothing more than revolutionary interlopers. The subversive corporeal acts of minorities, their infinite work of reappropriation, of resignification or cultural translation, terms which we find in works penned by Butler, never sufficiently shatter either the *logos* or the capitalist marketplace. Despite the contortions and the stylistic devices, despite multiplied identities and reiterated gestures, the rhetorical, pantomimical, and spectral represent much ado about nothing. They do not reinvent what speaking means. "The postmodern emergence of new multiple political subjectivities certainly does not reach this radical level of the political act proper."[34]

On the contrary, such radicality would be at work in the analytical act, on the condition that the latter relies on the real. Such an act would prove to be the only act capable of shattering all the configurations – including the economic – that structure the discourse of the subject. For Žižek, this act depends upon and revalorizes the unavoidable difference between the sexes.

> Lacan allows for a much more radical subjective intervention than Butler: what the Lacanian notion of "act" aims at is not a mere displacement/resignification of the symbolic coordinates that confer on the subject his or her identity, but the radical transformation of the very universal structuring "principle" of the existing symbolic order.[35]

Žižek's assault disturbs gender trouble. It is true that gender extends the list of actions, identities, possible ways of life but, at bottom, it does not manage to deeply reconfigure the impossibility upon which each and every life is based.

The *queer* would very much like to break with the duality of the sexes, in so doing they would wind up taking action, in the wake of which society would be fundamentally transformed, a truly radically revolutionary act. Their grievances are substantial, and they are here blamed for wanting to lead an armchair revolution. Between the comfort of university campuses and the precarity of large cities where their anger is manifest, the *queer* bubble, as light as it is brilliant, with its shifting and shimmering colours, only inflates in order to burst without managing to tarnish world affairs. Worse yet, this movement is only inflated with neo-liberal air, air born of an ultra-individualist and hyper-linguistic postmodernism. In a paradoxical manner, it is almost as if, the postmodern or deconstructivist postmodernism, having been applied to the body, found itself obliged to repudiate sexual difference. And, in so doing, found itself incapable of fighting in a concrete manner, from the standpoint of the reality of what we are, against the most fundamental dominations: those that are the result of economic materialism, of the structural hierarchies of our society, of the unjust systems inscribed within patriarchy, of mass consumerism, and of gender and class inequalities. The *queer* twist and turn, they perform, they thwart *straight* eroticism in detaching themselves from the duality of the sexes. They critique the patriarchal, oppressive, normative, heterocentric society. They mock it, they parody it. But, in so doing, they lose sight of their bodies in the course of their struggle. But this oversight prevents them from fully transvaluating the capitalist dynamics and their attachment to the *ego consummans*. Significantly, they unceasingly aspire to greater inclusivity, to the recognition of ever more rights, to the consideration of their humanity, of their differences and their specificities.[36] In this manner, while showing deep contempt for the reality of the sexes, they are quite determined to want to be accepted for what they are, individually, in the world as it is. Žižek thus asks "is there not always one struggle which, although it appears to function as one in the series, effectively provides the horizon of the series as such?"[37] This horizon would be that which would have left behind those who too rapidly embraced even the most left wing, poststructuralist lines of reasoning.

> They never question the fundamentals of the capitalist market economy and the liberal-democratic political regime; they never envisage the possibility of a completely different economico-political regime. In this way, they fully participate in the abandonment of these questions by the "postmodern" Left: all the changes they propose are changes within this economico-political regime.[38]

Butler approaches the real

I would like, on one hand, to respond to the perhaps overhasty accusation that Butler mistakes psychoanalytic subversion in so far as she takes inadequate account of what it is all about in actual fact; on the other it is important to me to show how the conception of *queer* sexualities and subjectivities, all while calling the preconceptions of *the* difference between the sexes into question, and while having arisen in the neoliberal context, are no less marked by an extreme interest in deconstructing the inequalities linked to patriarchy, class, and race. In short, more than a mere limitation of *queer*,

Butler seizes upon this polemic in order to complexify a line of thought that sees itself as radically leftist, well away from the hedonist temptation that is proper to hyper-industrial capitalism.[39] Furthermore, understanding the manner in which Butler appropriates the Lacanian real is of a double advantage for psychoanalysts: freeing them from both the reification of desire as from that of the real. Suffice it to say that, after having examined this debate with the real, the psychoanalytic clinic could pride itself on advancing a micropolitical valency when faced with the standardization of subjectivities. Moreover, the "case-by-case" approach to which it lays claim would no longer be confounded with a undefined mass individualism where each and every one selfishly pursues their own reductive happiness. Finally, and in a completely *queer* manner, this could perhaps open up a path for us, leading to that which could be signified beyond *the* difference between the sexes. Within the context of the clinic, the *queer* would no longer testify to an abstraction and to a universalization of desire, but to the manner in which the emergence of a real, singular in every occasion, revives the conditions whereby work on the construction of a desire which lies beyond norms is possible.

It is essential to understand that the consideration of the real in Lacan, as in Žižek and Butler, constitutes a manner of situating oneself not only outside the snare of nature and of biology, but also outside the snare of the symbolic and of culture at the precise moment when the question regarding *the* difference between the sexes is posed. This difference, once envisaged from the standpoint of the real, which has already been the subject of our interest in our aforementioned reading of Lacan's seminar XX, should no longer be understood as a purely physical difference nor as a purely signified one.

In *Giving an Account of Oneself* Butler identifies two ways of practicing psychoanalysis. The first is more psychologizing, conservative even, we could clearly identify it as acting in a major key. It is forged through the analyses of Paul Ricoeur and would occupy itself in making the account of oneself an organization, well-regulated and definitive, of who one is. To the completeness of such an account, Butler opposes a second version of psychoanalysis. The latter distances itself from the habitual version of analysis where the subject interweaves the strands of the past in order to attempt to make sense of their life.

> Indeed, some have argued that the normative goal of psychoanalysis is to permit the client to tell a single and coherent story about herself that will satisfy the wish to know herself, more-over, to know herself in part through a narrative reconstruction in which the interventions by the analyst or therapist contribute in many ways to the remaking and reweaving of the story.[40]

This is not a form of analysis that interests Butler. Without a doubt because she is still far too attached to the imaginary ties and the symbolic stakes. It is striking to note how Butler, to this initial version of psychoanalysis, opposes a question which seems to have been drawn from an introductory textbook on the clinic of the later Lacan:[41] "But what if the narrative reconstruction of a life cannot be the goal of psychoanalysis, and that the reason for this has to do with the very formation of the subject?"[42] Butler thus undertakes a demonstration of the construction of subjectivity where, given its attachment to something other than itself, by and through its inscription in the domain of the Other, the subject cannot, under any condition be limited to the Ego. It thus sees itself as fundamentally marked at once by both a void and by an excess that demolish even the most reassuring tentative to complete itself by means of narration. As a consequence, an ethical relation between the self, the other and the world is established. "The very possibility of linguistic agency is derived from the situation in which one finds oneself addressed by a language one never chose."[43]

Butler thereby reminds us in a precise manner of the stakes of an analytic cure that I would wholeheartedly qualify as being in a minor key:

> Full articulability should not be deemed the final goal of psychoanalytic work in any event, for that goal would imply a linguistic and egoic mastery over unconscious material that would seek to transform the unconscious itself into reflective, conscious articulation—an impossible ideal, and one that undercuts one of the most important tenets of psychoanalysis. The "I" cannot knowingly fully recover what impels it, since its formation remains prior to its elaboration as reflexive self-knowing. This reminds us that conscious experience is only one dimension of psychic life, and that we cannot achieve by consciousness or language a full mastery over those primary relations of dependency and impressionability that form and constitute us in persistent and obscure ways.[44]

In this context, Butler begins to rethink transference. That is, the impossibility of completeness, at once for both subject and for language itself, leads the construction of transference. "If the transference recapitulates the unconscious, then I undergo a dispossession of myself in the scene of address. This does not mean that I am possessed by the other, since the other is also dispossessed, called upon, and calling, in a relation that is not, for that reason, reciprocal."[45]

The inaccessibility of the origin determines the impossibility of narration which comes to a successful end. It works towards transferential movements: from this point a fantasy emerges and is constructed. The latter is formed so as to face the mystery of origin. The moment when one disentangles oneself from the myth of the fully constituted Ego, due to the original gulf that cannot be sutured and through which it is constituted, a fantasmic dimension appears as a response to the real. The real is the void, vacuous, the yawning gap which haunts each and every one of our remarks in their repetitive impetus in order to veil this exclusion that lies within discourse itself. This inalterable remainder is consistent with the weight of its own vacuousness. That is what each subject comes to question in the course of their cure. Like it or not, Butler here transcribes Lacan's aphorism in her own words: "the subject [...] is response to the real."[46] In fact, the dependence upon the Other, as well as the gaping hole in the foundation of the narrative of the self, are themselves rooted in the mystery of our own sexual origin, whatever it may have been. The attachment to a lineage that precedes us – even the queerest of lineages – implies a connection to the Other and, thus, signals the evident absence of any and all self-conception. Because I am not born of myself, I depend upon the Other. And because I depend upon the other, I suffer from a lack of completeness within my Ego. This enigmatic lack compels me to set up a long series of fantasmic hypotheses which help me to face the absence of coherence entailed by sexuality that, in its simplest form, anchors itself in the reproduction of the species.[47]

Thus read, Butler deploys an argumentation that is extremely close to that which we read in the later Lacan.

There is no sexual relationship

In turn, Žižek more strenuously underlines the fact that the subject, as response to the real, is first faced with Lacan's formula, little used by Butler, whereby "there is no sexual relationship." This refers, first and foremost, to the incompleteness at once of the subject and of language. There is another way to understand the well-known phrase "there is no meta-language" that is often uttered by structuralists: there is no point from which an overview of language as it deploys itself can be gained. When it comes down to it, and contrary to what biology, mathematics, formal logic, grand philosophical systems, and even structuralist linguistics, aspire to, "there is no" between human beings, quite simply.

This void, this absence, this failure, this point of foreclosing turns out to be necessary so as to set language itself in motion. Escaping from all realities, it renders them all possible in all possible variations. The "there is no sexual relationship" marks the point of incompleteness of all subjects and all discourses. Its inscription in the life of our bodies *and* in the symbolic field favours the constructions, the differences, the historicity through which our genders, our bodies and our sexualities can be expressed. "It thus seems more productive to posit as the central enigma that of sexual difference – not as the already established symbolic difference (heterosexual normativity) but, precisely, as that which forever eludes the grasp of normative symbolization."[48]

According to Žižek's reading of the later Lacan, the absence of the sexual relationship allows us to read *the* difference between the sexes in a new light. It is dedramatized. It is deprived of its normative dimension in aid of a sort of a condition of possibility which mars the universal characteristic of self-affirmative logic.

> Sexual difference is the Real of an antagonism, not the Symbolic of a differential opposition: sexual difference is not the opposition allocating to each of the two sexes its positive identity defined in opposition to the other sex (so that woman is what man is not, and vice versa), but a common Loss on account of which woman is never fully a woman and man is never fully a man – "masculine" and "feminine" positions are merely two modes of coping with this inherent obstacle/loss.[49]

This conception of the Lacanian real is particularly stimulating: in not renouncing the self-evident dualism that there are either men, or women, this conception concedes nothing as concerns a positivist or essentialist content that would amount to the realization of a possible masculine or feminine nature. On the contrary, the real becomes the obstacle which sets discourse in motion towards its own enigma. Žižek does not stop there. He attempts to definitively respond to the homophobic suspicions that weigh on Lacan seen as the unremitting defender of the symbolic law. "It is the very focus on the notion of Real as impossible that reveals the ultimate contingency, fragility (and thus changeability) of every symbolic constellation that pretends to serve as the a priori horizon of the process of symbolization."[50] In which case, the Law, the Father, the Phallus or Oedipus are seen as systematically pluralized. Relying on the familial or social norms in order to illustrate universality would reveal itself to be an error of logic.

Thus manifested, the Lacanian real is a powerful weapon which counters the psychoanalytic limits that the American philosopher has striven to contain in *Gender Trouble.* Žižek has thus understood Butler's criticisms concerning an overly structuralist version of the human psyche. His insistence upon the importance of the real and his approach to *the* difference from the standpoint of the absence of the sexual relationship testify to this. Rigidifying the law of the symbolic equates to oppressing the minorities. And yet, according to Žižek, Lacanian psychoanalysis has at its disposal an ethics and an act that is subversive in a wholly other manner.

> For Lacan, sexual difference is not a firm set of "static" symbolic oppositions and inclusions/exclusions (heterosexual normativity which relegates homosexuality and other "perversions" to some secondary role), but the name of a deadlock, of a trauma, of an open question, of something that resists every attempt at its symbolization.[51]

In other words, the Lacanian subject is fundamentally barred. This is not under any circumstances reducible to a normative or social exclusion. Whatever your preference, you will be barred, marked by the void, by a radical exclusion, an excess without name that will haunt your body marked by language even if you are of the most irreproachable heterosexuality. An excess of the real, an obscene surplus, an inevitable cock up lies in the hollow of every symbolic construction, whatever its orientation. One thereby escapes from the temptations of universalism, of uniformization, or of *a priori* ontological rejection. Foreclosure, the hole, the bar, the less than, the "there is no," liberate the horizons of each and every one, free to sketch themselves out as they see fit, independent from any consideration of the social, imaginary, or even the symbolic.

Reification in every gender

All of that is very good and well. Such a description of our conditions of possibility through which we can affirm what we are from the starting point of our bodies and our inscription in the field of the Other proves to be, in fact, particularly ethical. The incompleteness tears a hole in our certitudes and allows everyone to invent their own way of expressing themselves in speech. Owing to the absence of the sexual relationship, we would be ever so close to the truth at the very moment when we prepare ourselves to take leave of the notion of truth itself. What more is there to say on this from a *queer* point of view? Can we rejoice in having found in this text the possibility of, at last, reconciling gender deconstruction with psychoanalysis or, better yet, perhaps the absence of the sexual relationship is indicative of the *queerest* bit of psychoanalysis?[52]

Under these circumstances, the appeal to the real appears to offer a chance to escape from the impasses of psychoanalysis in a major key when it places too exclusive a trust in a signifying and heteronormative approach. The symbolic always runs the risk of being reified. It thus takes on the aspect of *the* absolute law incarnated by certain familial configurations to the exclusion of others. The real, once inscribed at the heart of the symbolic cuts short the overly ambitious thirst for conservative consistency. Thus, faced with so many pluralizations and openings, what more is there to say? What is there left to complain about? Why not savour in silence the intelligence and the perfection of the system spread open by the *nouage* of the symbolic the imaginary and the real? Why on earth must we still linger over the exalted grievances of a few minorities who have misunderstood the clarification of the repercussions of the real on our being?

It is because this appeal to the real, despite its ingenuity, resembles a meta-difference capable of organizing, uncentring the symbolic field and the social practices that arise out of it. Butler, strengthened by her alliances with sexual minorities, is astonished: does the trauma of the sexual within language, characterized by "there is no sexual relationship," impose itself forever and for all in the same way? Where does the efficiency of this description come from? Is this mechanism at work within all *parlêtres*? In what manner does this point of non-closure, un-suturable, line up with the political stakes? In paying heed to these questions, which are framed from the standpoint of sexual minorities, in place of the sole heterosexual reference as scaffold for thought, one drifts towards an approach to the real in a minor key.

Fundamentally, if Butler avoids referring to the real too often, it is not so much because she would not be well acquainted with its implications within the teachings of the later Lacan, but because therein she reads the trauma of the sexual, in and of language, as a prelude, an *a priori* condition, a logic which while certainly straining the universal, precedes the ideological interrogation of the manners in which the body can be experienced and described.

Thus, to say that Butler has not taken the real into account, is to heedlessly toil away. Even if references to the later seminars of Lacan do not abound in the pages she writes, she is not any less aware that the appeal to the real – so often present in the clinical texts of the most open Lacanians, including Žižek – unfolds not only ethical stakes (without a doubt opening up the notion of a case-by-case analysis and the singularity of each and every one) but also political stakes. To be quite clear, the question is the following: to what degree does the articulation of the Lacanian "there is no sexual relationship," which is meant to open the most ethical and subversive dimension of psychoanalysis, radicalizing the position of not-knowing, of suspense and surprise as a counterpoint to the logic of the universal and for all, to what degree is such a statement not, unknowingly, drawn from a radically heterosexual point of view? Has "there is no sexual relationship" not always, already and foremost, been considered from the standpoint of the heterosexual norm? Does this condition of the possibility of psychoanalytic thought, this transcendental ethics, not pronounce itself, as a matter of priority, in terms of there is no (hetero)sexual relationship? And, in this case, if the "there is no" refers to an exclusion beyond the sphere of what can be said, to what cannot be formulated, to a point of radical foreclosure that is characteristic of the apparition of the real directly within the symbolic, what aspects of reality, what forms of abnormal life have been vacuumed up by this vortex outside-of-sense?

In fact, the appeal to the real, as a condition of the possibility of psychoanalysis strongly resembles a manner of protecting oneself from relativist disorder. After the infinite structuralist differentiations and the post-structuralist relativizations, striving to deploy a logic of the real in order to buttress discourse, saves it from a culturalist chaos where everything goes. Without the real the world is unhinged. Without expressive impossibility, no formulations can test its logic. Of course, the real undermines universalist logic but in so doing it sets itself up as that which no one can escape. As inevitable as it may seem, Butler is wary of this line of reasoning. To her criticisms of the symbolic order as a law which structures humanity, it has been said that she has mistaken the real. Thus, orthodox Lacanians have delivered their final fatal blow to the *queer*:

> You are mistaken. You have made psychoanalysis into an old, conservative practice, incapable of taking living diversity into account. You have seen psychoanalysis as prescribing laws for all, in defence of the Oedipal and the patriarchy. But you have not seen that, in reality, its only beacon is the real. And this notion represents the negativity that inhabits every affirmation, the point of resistance that mars every advance in understanding. Such an unnameable impossibility inevitably imposes itself as the basis through which everybody is regulated. But nobody can escape from it. For all, forever, for all time and in all places, we differ: we are not subsumed to the same but to difference. Nevertheless, as we can see, admit it, each and every one encounters the necessity of the real, the necessity of a meta-point that is impossible to consider. There is no meta-discourse because there is no sexual relationship.

To which the *queer* answer back: "But, in this case, there is a meta-point of impossibility. A transcendental impossibility. You have reified the real."

The other side of the real

Butler may not have understood Lacan's theories. She may not have sufficiently understood the detail of the non-suturation of the symbolic by the real. She may not have knotted the link that binds the real, the symbolic, and the imaginary. Perhaps. But, in her dialogue with Žižek, her misunderstanding goes so far as to protect her from an immediate adhesion which would take the theory of the Lacanian real at face value. Or, in more favourable terms, it is without a doubt that Butler, indeed, and to begin with, did not perceive exactly what the real signifies. Nevertheless, as Žižek himself remarked concerning the reception of Derrida in the United States, it is possible that this misunderstanding of the Lacanian corpus highlights "its own 'repressed' truth."[53] Perhaps she has given the real occasion to be troubled by *the* difference between the sexes. In fact, from a minoritarian perspective, thinking through the failure of the sexual relationship between the sexes as the condition of the historicization of thought winds up orientating, in an exclusively heterosexual and binary manner, the stories that flow therefrom, and foreclosing those that do not conform thereto.

In "Arguing with the Real" in *Bodies that Matter*, Butler nevertheless aspires to the Outside. So for that thought to set itself in motion, it is evident that one must refer to the unthinkable. However, the philosopher refuses the absolutization of such an Outside. Its apparent conditions must properly be unceasingly renegotiated, rethought, reworked, in terms of its political and ethical consequences. This amounts to better circumscribing the contents of exclusion from whence each discursive formation draws its momentum. "But if we concur that every discursive formation proceeds through constituting an 'outside,' we are not thereby committed to the *invariant* production of that outside as the trauma of castration (nor to the generalization of castration as the model for all historical trauma)."[54] Quoting Žižek who himself refers to Hegel, she affirms that: "'the ultimate question is: which specific content has to be excluded so that the very empty form of universality emerges as the "battlefield" for hegemony?' And is it truly empty, or does it carry the trace of the excluded in spectral form as an internal disruption of its own formalism?"[55]

Should the real be taken into account as *the* ultimate condition of possibility for all differential movements? And can this condition of possibility comfortably superimpose itself upon *the* difference between the sexes? In this case, is one not dealing with a final effort, without a doubt subversive but nevertheless in a major key, to reintroduce invariability under the auspices of an inevitable failure? To what degree does the failure of the sexual relationship not find itself a home in a reality far more concrete and changing than in the forms of life that have been ignored, rejected, reduced to silence?

> The failure of every such unity can be reduced to a "lack" with no historicity, the consequence of a transhistorical "law," but such a reduction will miss the failures and discontinuities produced by social relations that invariably exceed the signifier and whose exclusions are necessary for the stabilization of the signifier. The "failure" of the signifier to produce the unity it appears to name is not the result of an existential void, but the result of that term's incapacity to include the social relations that it provisionally stabilizes through a set of contingent exclusions. This incompleteness will be the result of a specific set of social exclusions that return to haunt the claims of identity defined through negation.[56]

Earlier in the same text, Butler writes:

> That there is always an "outside" and, indeed, a "constitutive antagonism" seems right, but to supply the character and content to a law that secures the borders between the "inside" and the "outside" of symbolic intelligibility is to pre-empt the specific social and historical analysis that is required, to conflate into "one" law the effect of a convergence of many, and to preclude the very possibility of a future rearticulation of that boundary [...].[57]

The symbolic negation that is brought on by the real need not be recognized once and for all but should properly reach for the most extreme possibility. In no instance should it be assimilated to a unique fantasy, always already destined to fail, of the completeness of two, and only two, sexes, whether they be complementary, opposed, or even if their jouissances were to be designated as supplementary. Butler thus enjoins us to perceive how the dispossession of the Outside causes us to flee, pierces us, dislocates us beyond the heterocentrist matrix. Heteros, homos, trans, bi, *queer*, for each age of history, in accordance with the specific social, political, economic, and personal arrangements, it is incumbent upon us to take up the infinite task of rethinking the manner in which the Outside erodes us, displaces us, effaces us.

> Even if every discursive formation is produced through exclusion, that is not to claim that all exclusions are equivalent: what is needed is a way to assess politically how the production of cultural unintelligibility is mobilized variably to regulate the political field, i.e., who will count as a "subject," who will be required not to count. To freeze the real as the impossible "outside" to discourse is to institute a permanently unsatisfiable desire for an ever elusive referent: the sublime object of ideology. The fixity and universality of this relation between language and the real produces, however, a prepolitical pathos that precludes the kind of analysis that would take the real/reality distinction as the instrument and effect of contingent relations of power.[58]

For each subject, it amounts to accepting our ignorance as concerns the conditions of the emergence of our real. The exercise thus consists of identifying it, without too hastily returning to *the* difference between the sexes and without dispensing with the social conditions from whence the subject pronounces their discourse. Taking the real into account, is to take account of the complexity of its emergence: this is at the crossroads of the social, the political, the linguistic, and the intimate.

> That the term is questionable does not mean that we ought not to use it, but neither does the necessity to use it mean that we ought not perpetually to interrogate the exclusions by which it proceeds, and to do this precisely in order to learn how to live the contingency of the political signifier in a culture of democratic contestation.[59]

In not reifying the real, Butler lends her ear to the cacophony of the Outside. As Michel Foucault admirably formulated it in his homage to the literary work of Maurice Blanchot, "The pure outside of the origin, if that is indeed what language is eager to greet, never solidifies into a penetrable and immobile positivity."[60] By not fixing this Outside, by not absolutizing it, unceasingly rediscovering it and, in every instant opening one's eye to the manner in which exclusion, the impossibility to say everything, to put everything into words, forecloses the existence of other possibilities, other formulations.

"There is no recourse to a universal language, but neither is there recourse to a single structure or a single lack that underscores all discursive formations. Our exile in heterogeneity is, in this sense, irreversible."[61]

Thus, Žižek's insistence, in the wake of Lacan, on asserting the real of *the* difference between the sexes at once both outside the biological and the social as a "traumatic cut which disturbs the smooth functioning of the body [just like the] violence of the cultural 'transubstantiation' of the biological body through its sexuation"[62] does not prove to be sufficiently capable of accepting this exile within heterogeneity. The capacities for action too quickly see themselves as renewed within a binary and simplistic distribution between man/woman which, in seeking to suspend at once the weight of the norms, of language as well as that of biology, ends up reintroducing, by way of forgetting, the injustices, the precarities and the affronts which haunt the social. In other words, there where one would have thought to have relieved oneself of the invariable, one reproduces it, certainly as something which cannot be said, an Outside, a castration, unattainable, an internal limit of discourse, but one nevertheless reestablishes it as unavoidable, applicable to all *parlêtres* to the same degree.

Some clinical consequences

Envisaging the real from the standpoint of a minor key does not amount to recognizing the existence of a sexual relationship but amounts to reflecting on what prohibits, in an implicit manner, the inexistence of this relationship. Such a relationship has, firstly, been considered from the standpoint of the division of the two sexes who sought, in vain, to complete each other. In other words, the "there is no sexual relationship" was elaborated within a matrix which renders discourse heteronormative. That is not, for all that, to say that there is a homosexual relationship. Nor does this mean that any success in such a relationship could take place in the field of sexual minorities. On the contrary, this drives the exploration of that which is implicit in the appeal to the real which is the sole and unique beacon, representing an *a priori* reflex, a buttress which sustains reflection, a support in the accomplishment of what would be an authentic act. Even though *the* difference between the sexes certainly plays an important role in our manner of envisaging that which can and cannot be thought, it is our right to question ourselves regarding the manner in which its use, and its identification with the real has a political effect upon those who do not directly recognize themselves therein and who nevertheless feel traumatized in every instant of their lives on account of who they are! Are these subjects directly representative of the unthinkable? If this is the case, one would exclude from reality, in the name of the real, a certain number of people who, nevertheless exist in the flesh! Should the appeal to the real of *the* difference between the sexes serve only to, once again, relegate these subjects to silence?

Butler's perspective demands more strenuous consideration of the minor spaces wherein the dominant discourse and its epistemology is contested. We are not, here, engaged in an inclusive exercise or in the broadening of the field of possibilities from the standpoint of gender relativism. Rather, we value the different manners of access to the impossibility of jouissance. The sexual minorities, in so far as they are on the front lines of unbearable realities – realities of insult, humiliation, relegation to legal exclusion and to silence – set us on the path of another access to the real. The stakes lie not in the pluralisation of the Name-of-the-Father, as Lacan judiciously proposed in the beginning of the 60s,[63] but in the complexification of our modes of representation of the internal void that is characteristic of each subject and of the Other. Given that their inconsistence was at first conceptualized through a *straight* unthought, in a heteronormative silence, through an unsaid that proves itself to be brutal for all those who do not immediately recognize themselves in this reflexive matrix, much remains to be done.

In the absence of this effort of reconceptualization, the real as impossible to address remains, always and forever, the foundation of the political regulation of bodies: an alibi in order to continue to distinguish normal from pathological on the same basis. The stakes are not exclusively theoretical, political, and ethical, they are also clinical. They imply the pathologization of those who do not feel an evident alignment with the binarity of gender. In the light of this "argument with the real" one sees that the call, even transcendental to *the* difference between the sexes has too often a tendency to flirt with a sort of return of the domination of women by men, of homosexuals by heterosexuals. The stakes lie in the social repercussions of the analytic dispositive itself: does its existence perpetuate inequalities, or does it contribute to a perspective that allows one to better oppose said inequalities?

Adieu to the gods

I am not seeking to deny the existence of *the* probable difference between the sexes. I do not want to upset, at any cost, our self-evident perception so as to thwart certain pillars of psychoanalytic theory. But it seems necessary to me to question oneself on the implications of an account of the psyche exclusively seen through this binarism. More precisely, is it indispensable to raise this tricky subject which strives to scamper off when faced with such preconceptions? Why is there such an attachment to the duality of the sexes?

Because psychoanalytic work reflects on the status of our being, composed of flesh and of words, of sex and of language, of drives and sublimations; because it aims to propel becoming without guaranteeing its accomplishment, without any certitude as to its realization, without preconceptions concerning the constructions and the momentum that it leads to; in short, because psychoanalytic work de-constructs, dis-places, un-knots, such an exercise cannot content itself with *the* difference between the sexes as a simple mask for the hierarchy where One imposes its diktat upon the Other.

With her supposed misunderstanding of the appeal to the real, Butler recognizes the shift from the anatomical to the categorical. She aids the psychoanalytic clinic in no longer supporting, for better or for worse, the *status quo* of inequalities between men and women.

To better understand the manner in which theory, politics, ethics, and the clinical are intertwined around this appeal to consider a beyond *the* difference between the sexes as a sole and unique reference for the apprehension of the real, a reading of *Sexing the Body* by Anne Fausto-Sterling is invaluable. This consideration, half-way between the history of biology and that of feminism extends the paths opened up by *Gender Trouble*. It offers the opportunity to reread the teachings of Lacan from, what at the very least, can be described as a *queer* viewpoint.

In exhaustively going through the conflicts of differing scientific theories elaborated regarding *the* difference between the sexes and the incoherencies that have spurred them on for nearly a century, Fausto-Sterling shows how sex, before even being a biological or anatomical fact, possesses a political determination. At times considering the question of hormones, while at other times concentrating on the question of chromosomes, considering the manipulation of genes, or in observing the brain, or even studying rats and mice, researchers have applied themselves in circumscribing the location in which *the* difference between man and woman can be situated. Articles, publications, scientific discoveries, and declarations in the quest for an indubitable sexual authenticity have unceasingly rewoven the mystery of this difference, testifying to the difficulty in sifting true from false as concerns this subject.

The scientific discoveries prove to be irremediably situated in a given place and time. Despite the interest that they hold, they are guilty of a certain lack of neutrality. Whatever the objective pretentions of research, its knowledge proves to be partially located in a partisan way. For Anne Fausto-Sterling, these experiments do not follow on from one another in the coldly rigorous manner that is expected of the laboratory understood in the light of a happily teleology of progress. They are but the reflections of political stakes and struggles. Each analysis that undergoes her careful reading ultimately betrays a dualist prejudice, at once heteronormative and hierarchical… The quotidian practice of science involves itself in "social belief systems […] in ways that are often invisible to the working scientist."[64] Most of the time, the interpretation of the results obtained only serves to confirm cultural preconceptions that are orientated by the biologists' starting point. Fausto-Sterling does not mince her words: "labeling someone a man or a woman is a social decision. We may use scientific knowledge to help us make the decision, but only our beliefs about gender—not science—can define our sex."[65] Further on in her work she explains that our bodies are too anatomically complex to offer cut and dry answers to the question of *the* difference between the sexes. What effect does this new deconstruction of *the* difference between the sexes have regarding psychoanalysis?

It is interesting to note that Fausto-Sterling, with the help of a text by Elisabeth Grosz, develops her reflection in considering the Möbius band. This topological figure also plays a decisive role in Lacan's teaching. On this strange ribbon, the interior and the exterior are no longer opposed but belong to the same surface in perpetual torsion. When we follow along the band we unceasingly pass from the outside inside and vice versa. This figure illustrates the regression of an analysis where one passes from the conscious to the unconscious, from the said to the unsaid, from idle talk to a crucial detail. According to Lacan, "the subject has the structure of a surface at least topologically defined."[66] For Anne Fausto-Sterling, this figure represents the constant passage between the social and the biological. In one instance as in the other, the two aspects of the same path are drawn gradually as one progresses. The trajectory proposed by Fausto-Sterling moves from the exterior of the body toward the interior and then outwards again. In step with what Butler develops in *Gender Trouble*, Fausto-Sterling considers that the binarism of gender has influenced studies which seek to divide the sexes into two airtight biological categories. The same can be said for what lies beyond this, that is to say the social, the connections that each living person encounters in the course of their life, and which give consistence to the materiality of their bodies.

To the binarity of the sexes, Fausto-Sterling prefers a "continuum of sexes" as extensive as the colours of a refractive prism.

> While male and female stand on the extreme ends of a biological continuum, there are many other bodies [...] that evidently mix together anatomical components conventionally attributed to both males and females. The implications of my argument for a sexual continuum are profound. If nature really offers us more than two sexes, then it follows that our current notions of masculinity and femininity are cultural conceits.[67]

One should not however read Fausto-Sterling's text as a plea in favour of a relativism in which anything and everything could be said regarding our bodies, but rather as written in praise of complexity and diversity: the complexity and diversity of our bodies and our beings, the complexity and diversity of the real, the complexity and diversity of sociological, biological, and metapsychological approaches. Each and every time, there is no other goal than the perpetual destabilization of that which is considered as "normal." For Fausto-Sterling, gender, like sex is neither individual, nor private, nor fixed, but in perpetual interaction, under permanent construction, and never definitively established.[68]

Staking out a position of this nature within the field of biology is rare and invaluable. It extends the domain of possibilities in offering new viewpoints. This "argument with the real" allows us to envisage minoritarian resistance, no longer seen as merely the demands of identitarian splinter groups, themselves determined by oppositions of signification to which they must give consistency in order to make themselves heard, but rather from the standpoint of the conception of what being confronted with a jouissance and a real outside-of-sense can signify. It thus amounts to experiencing the spectre of multiplicities that engender the ab-sense sex. In other words, how can we consider the real beyond *the* difference between the sexes? Well, back to the drawing board and Lacan's tables of sexuation!

Queer sexuation

Lacan's table of sexuation can be read in a major key. While he profoundly frustrates the propositional oppositions of the Aristotelian square of opposition, he reproduces *the* difference between the sexes. This difference is herein envisaged neither in terms of anatomy nor in terms of the symbolic but from the standpoint of the real of jouissance as a fundamental non-relationship. By means of this failure, as we have seen, two types of jouissance see the light of day. From this point, how can we use the table of sexuation if, instead of privileging *the* difference between the sexes, we take the path of the continuum of the sexes? Can we push his manner of disrupting the order of the said even further so as to better account for the multiplicities of the said? In superimposing the real of jouissance upon the findings of Fausto-Sterling, can we seize upon the table and formulas of sexuation as of a hitherto unseen performative occasion, that is truly in a minor key?

In *On Feminine Sexuality, the Limits of Love and Knowledge*, Lacan does not procrastinate any more than Fausto-Sterling: "biological metaphors clearly cannot reassure us here – they reassure us here still less than elsewhere."[69] There is no comfort in the biological, which is of little assurance. The so-called laws of nature, the anatomical pseudo self-evidences, the biological functions, even if considered as images or metaphors are insufficiently able to offer a rationale regarding what we are as subjects inhabited by language and haunted by the real of jouissance. In fact, as Fausto-Sterling remarks,

> There are hormones, genes, prostates, uteri, and other body parts and physiologies that we use to differentiate male from female, that become part of the ground from which varieties of sexual experience and desire emerge. Furthermore, variations in each of these aspects of physiology profoundly affect an individual's experience of gender and sexuality.[70]

But these material elements and innumerable contradictions of different medical and scientific analytic protocols that have attempted to assure a vague stability have nevertheless testified to "the insistent complexity of actual bodies and personalities."[71] It is all very well and good to aspire to a unequivocable explanation of these variations, however the body refuses to cooperate. "Every time we try to return to the body as something that exists prior to socialization, prior to discourse about male and female, Butler writes, 'we discover that matter is fully sedimented with discourses on sex and sexuality that prefigure and constrain the uses to which that term can be put.'"[72]

Lacan is thus clairvoyant when he turns away from biology and approaches the question of jouissance. "The discourse of analysis differs from scientific discourse."[73] Encountering the unconscious means putting scientific pretentions to truth in their place. What he discovered in Aristotle, the valiant logician of Being and of meaning, was one of his first champions. We thus enter the zone of discomfort and of paradoxes that the truth and its aspirations to the universality of the concept can do nothing other than spoil. Beginning with Freud's discovery, "reality is approached with the apparatuses of jouissance."[74] This is another way of expressing Freud's famous and cruel vexation:

> that the life of our sexual instincts cannot be wholly tamed, and that mental processes are in themselves unconscious and only reach the ego and come under its control through incomplete and untrustworthy perceptions – these two discoveries amount to a statement that the ego is not master in its own house.[75]

An earthquake in the realm of knowledge. Even the most noble of abstractions do little more than hide our misery: "If analytic discourse indicates that that meaning is sexual, that can only be by explaining its limit. [...] Meaning (*sens*) indicates the direction toward which it fails (*échoue*)."[76] Biology and philosophy are of no assurance when faced with the real of jouissance: "the sexual relationship drops into the abyss of nonsense."[77] Lacan later adds that "the whole truth is what cannot be told. It is what can only be told on the condition that one doesn't push it to the edge, that one only half-tells (*mi-dire*) it."[78] For all that, psychoanalytic discourse does not abandon the notion that it works in a scientific manner. It makes "science [...] of the real."[79] This science retraces the place of desire, not so much as from *the* difference between the sexes, understood as an anatomical law, as a "corporeal contingency."[80] Writing the quantifiers of the table of sexuation furnishes "a medium (*support*) that goes beyond speech, without going beyond language's actual effects."[81] Lacan's antiphilosophy thus does not consist of refuting the history of the truth, of language games, of being and of meaning but in allowing oneself to be traversed by these from the position of incompleteness, the yawning gap, the "there is no."[82]

What is more, the table of sexuation asserts a logical quantifier other than those forged by the Aristotle, the Stagirite and his disciples: the "not whole." Its quantification localizes a space representing an exception: a jouissance, which for Lacan is *a priori* feminine, which would call into question the universalist quest for meaning, typically masculine and phallic, all the while rendering it possible. "It's peculiar that it's only with the analytic discourse that a universal can find its veritable fundament in the existence of an exception. At any rate, this means that we can certainly distinguish the universal that is founded from any use that is rendered commonplace by the philosophical tradition of the said universal."[83] The "for all" which is the marker of phallic masculine jouissance and its inscription in the cogs of language, is contradicted by the "not whole." Nevertheless, it is clear that women are inscribed to the left of the table beneath the category of "for all." Certain powerful women, certain hysterics are able to align themselves with the phallic regime. Further on in his seminar, Lacan confirms this anatomical relativization with regard to jouissance itself:

> when one is male [...] one can also situate oneself on the side of the not-whole. There are men who are just as good as women. It happens. And who also feel just fine about it. Despite – I won't say their phallus – despite what encumbers them that goes by that name, they get the idea or sense that there must be a jouissance that is beyond.[84]

Thus, the so-called feminine part of the table remains inaccessible to either sex, whatever their anatomy. "Any speaking being whatsoever, as is expressly formulated in Freudian theory, whether provided with the attributes of masculinity – attributes that remain to be determined – or not, is allowed to inscribe itself in this part."[85] Having left the "un-wholly" phallic logic behind, as applicable to all, anatomy is no longer indicative of anything at all, not even the distinction that relegates one to the Other, the unavowable, the informulable. Here the proud attributes of masculinity, those who preside over the phallogocentrism of the philosophical tradition, are themselves indetermined. This opens up a veritable gender freedom which, more precisely, throws the pretentions to truth of language and of anatomy off balance.

Nevertheless, Lacan only successfully completes four formulas of sexuation. Does his breakthrough, moving beyond the logical exercise of language from the starting point of a quadrangle, finally intersect with dualism? If the answer to this question were to be in the affirmative, we would be off to a bad start in our desire to lend an ear to bodies such as they express themselves and live their lives today. How to move past the strict repartition of Lacan's table of sexuation so as to place emphasis not on *the* difference between the sexes but on the (multiple) "*contingencies* of bodies"? If Lacan lands a blow aimed at both Aristotle and occidental metaphysics, is it not possible for us to aim a blow at him, on behalf of the oppressed minorities and through the work of Fausto-Sterling? Beyond a reading in a major key of the table which can serve to reinterpret the limits of Freud's aphorism "anatomy is destiny,"[86] can we offer a reading in a minor key? This second reading would strain the universal, multiply the positions right up until they grab hold of us and unify us, not from the standpoint of that which is identical, but through our differences. Well away from the universally abstract constants, and as close as can be to the real of jouissance, a new form of logic begins to see the light of day.

In a short but provocative and ironic conference which has attracted quite a measure of attention, Anne Fausto-Sterling proposed the existence of not two but five sexes![87] "In addition to males and females, I argued, we should also accept the categories herms (named after 'true' hermaphrodites), merms (named after male 'pseudo-hermaphrodites'), and ferms (named after female 'pseudo-hermaphrodites')."[88] In so doing Fausto-Sterling not only came to the defence of a queer radical relativism but also to that of children born intersex – not quite as rare an occurrence as one would imagine (representing 1.7% of births) where a child is born with genital organs that are midway between that of a girl or a boy. These newborns are still too often submitted to genital aesthetic and surgical sexual reassignation procedures which aim to obtain their adequation with one of the two sexes.[89] In her article the biologist explains: "Hermaphrodites have unruly bodies. They do not fall naturally into a binary classification, only a surgical shoehorn can put them there."[90] The violence of the treatment that has been inflicted upon this practically invisible and inaudible minority of subjects born intersex, makes blindingly obvious "a cultural need to maintain clear distinctions between the sexes. Society mandates the control of intersexual bodies because they blur and bridge the great divide. Inasmuch as hermaphrodites literally embody both sexes, they challenge traditional beliefs about sexual difference: they possess the irritating ability to live sometimes as one sex and sometimes the other, and they raise the spectre of homosexuality."[91] Of course a society in which we would recognize five sexes instead of two would be a utopia. Fausto-Sterling's proposition requires an effort of imagination. She pins her hopes on a renewed ethics: "Imagine that the sexes have multiplied beyond currently imaginable limits. It would have to be a world of shared powers. Patient and physician, parent and child, male and female, heterosexual and homosexual – all those oppositions and other would have to be dissolved as sources of division."[92] This utopia should not be confused with a return to an ideal of completeness in whatever form it may take. It does not amount to fulfilling, through the multiplication of genders and sexes, the incompleteness of our bodies. Rather, it amounts to no longer limiting division to a hierarchical binarism that always already implies *the* difference between the sexes. The prism of the continuum of the sexes does not deny diversity, but no longer determines it in terms of *the* difference.

In his table of sexuation, Lacan squared off the two sexes. He arrives at four formulas. And if we were to follow the provocative course laid out by Fausto-Sterling? And if we squared off the five sexes? This would give rise to no less than twenty-five formulas of sexuation! The table of the modes of jouissance would thus reduce the rigour of the Aristotelian formulation to dust. The square of opposition which thus results from this exercise would be just about irrepresentable. It would preclude any belief in the linearity that is characteristic of the development of formal logic and its rigorous oppositions. It would definitively ruin the "for all." The affirmation of the real of jouissance as being "not whole" would find itself multiplied. The corporeal contingencies would be able to pinpoint themselves, being able to express, each in their own way, the failure of the sexual. In this manner, we would continue to "have recourse to the not-all (*pastout*) […] in other words to the impasses of logic."[93] One would leave the mythic dualist fictions behind so as to "make of the real a different fixion"[94] that is, to understand on a case-by-case basis for all, "the impossibility that affixes it to the structure of language. Which also means tracing the path through which, in each discourse, the real in which it is wrapped up is found, and dismissing the myths with which it is ordinarily supplemented."[95] What does this mean exactly? That the homophonic thickness that makes Lacan's writing so complex enjoins us to unceasingly renew the meaning of his writing. That to fixate oneself on the dualism of *the* difference throws us into the realm of fiction, cultural but unfounded, rather than to that of fixion where meaning, proper to each and every one is fixed. In "L'étourdit" Lacan reminds us, in French that "*deux*" (two) is equivocal: it can also be written and heard as "*d'eux*" (of them).[96]

Let us move from *deux* to *d'eux*. Who are "*d'eux*"? And how do they fail in the sexual relationship? In 1997, in her first visit to France, and in the course of an international conference on "Gay and Lesbian Studies" at the Centre Georges Pompidou, Eve Kosofsky Sedgwick proposed a definition of *queer* politics. She recounted "the number and *difference* of the dimensions that 'sexual identity' is supposed to organize into a seamless and univocal whole."[97] To rally the *queer* is to accept the senseless that systematically brings the compact univocality of the totality to failure. In other words, it is to moor oneself to the "not whole." It is abandoning the classical representations of the subject in order to perceive the mobile and plural constitution of our subjectivities. Will Fausto-Sterling's five sexes, squared off in Lacan's logic, be enough to embrace that which the word *queer* can refer to: "lapses, and excesses of meaning when the constituent elements of anyone's gender, of anyone's sexuality aren't made (or can't be made) to signify monolithically"?[98] In lending an ear to the equivocal side of signification, the monoliths are reduced to dust. *Deux* becomes *d'eux*. Within the boxing ring, the *queers* and the psychoanalysts combat each other, oppose each other, superimpose upon one another, embrace one another. And twenty-five positions of jouissance trace

> the experimental linguistic, epistemological, representational, political adventures, attaching to the very many of us who may at times be moved to describe ourselves as (among many other possibilities) pushy femmes, radical faeries, fantasists, *drags, clones*, leatherfolk, ladies in tuxedos, feminist women or feminist men, masturbators, bulldaggers, divas, *Snap*! Queens, butch bottoms, storytellers, transsexuals, aunties, wannabes, lesbian-identified men, or lesbians who sleep with men, or ... people able to relish, learn from, or identify with *such*.[99]

This inventory defaces the consistency of all masks. In its own way, it renews with the plasticity of the drive, the polymorphic nature of Freudian sexuality. Conscious of the irreducibility of the incompleteness, it turns away from that which hides *deux* in order to hear and understand that which is said in every manner and by every gender, as from *d'eux*.

In effacing *the* difference between the sexes "like a face drawn in sand at the edge of the sea"[100] one does not dismiss, with a wave of the hand, the psychoanalytic motor. Quite the contrary. The peal of bodies continues to sound out, in the light of the impossibility of the relationship. Eros and Thanatos unceasingly embrace. In these spaces, float the nebulous complexes wherein no one is sheltered from hesitation, ambiguity, and enigma. The eddies swamp the certitudes. The waves carry along that which must be, and that which is legitimate in a perpetual movement of backwash. Senses succumb to the real. Jouissance unfurls. And on the horizon, desire erupts into view. Such a shore is always in a state of evolution. Its contours cry out for a perpetual reproblematization. "Birth and death, and the difference between the sexes, are the complex themes of problems before they are the simple terms of an opposition. [...] It may be that there is necessarily something mad in every question and every problem, as there is in their transcendence in relation to answers, in their insistence through solutions and in the manner in which they maintain their own openness."[101] It is with this madness that it is necessary to continue to traverse the expanses of thought and of the clinic in a minor key.

Notes

1 This is the explicit position of Charles Melman, "Édito," *Le Bulletin Lacanien 4: "Sex and gender"* (Association Lacanienne internationale, 2008), 9.
2 Tim Dean, "Lacan and queer theory" in *The Cambridge Companion to Lacan*, ed. Jean-Michel Rabaté (Cambridge University Press, 2003), 247.
3 Sigmund Freud, "Beyond the Pleasure Principle" in *The Standard Edition of the Complete Psychological Works of Sigmund Freud*. Vol. XVIII. Edited by James Strachey, Anna Freud, and Angela Richards. (Hogarth Press, 1953 - 1974), 1–64.

4 Jacques Lacan, *The Four Fundamental Concepts of Psychoanalysis. The Seminar of Jacques Lacan. Book XI 1963–1964*, ed. Jacques-Alain Miller, trans. Alan Sheridan (W.W. Norton & Company, 1978).
5 "[…] réapparaît dans le coprs, dans n'importe quelle partie où existait un passage entre l'intérier et l'extérieur." Javier Saez, *Théorie queer et psychanalyse* (EPEL, 2005), 35.
6 This expression is drawn from an unpublished seminar, *Extimité*, that was given by Jacques-Alain Miller in the Psychoanalysis Department of the University of Paris 8 in the 1985–1986 school year. It is available online here: https://jonathanleroy.be/wp-content/uploads/2016/01/1985-1986-Extimité-JA-Miller.pdf
7 Tim Dean, "Lacan and queer theory" in *The Cambridge Companion to Lacan*, ed. Jean-Michel Rabaté (Cambridge University Press, 2003), 249.
8 "Le fait que l'objet *a* soit indépendant du genre (il n'est ni masculine, ni féminin) permettra d'établin une lecture non hétérocentrée de la psychanalyse." Javier Saez, *Théorie queer et psychanalyse* (EPEL, 2005), 35.
9 Jacques Lacan, *On Feminine Sexuality, The Limits of Love and Knowledge. The Seminar of Jacques Lacan. Book XX*, ed. Jacques-Alain Miller, trans. Bruce Fink (W.W. Norton & Company, 1998), 66.
10 Jacques Lacan, *The Ethics of Psychoanalysis, The Seminar of Jacques Lacan. Book VII 1959–1960*, ed. Jacques-Alain Miller, trans. Dennis Porter (Routledge, 1992).
11 See Jacques Lacan, "L'étourdit" in Autres Écrits (Seuil, 2001), 449–497. This text has been partially translated in Jacques Lacan, "L'étourdit" *The Letter* 41, trans. Cormac Gallagher, (2009), 31–80.
12 Jacques Lacan, "L'étourdit" *The Letter*, 32.
13 "Un dire extérieur au di test appelé à l'existence par l'intermédiaire du l'entendu; un *dire* extérieur à l'entendu est appelé à l'existence par l'intermédiaire du dit." Christian Fierens, *Lecture de L'étourdit. Lacan 1972* (L'Harmattan, 2002), 42.
14 Jacques Lacan, "L'étourdit" *The Letter*, 38.
15 Jacques Lacan, "L'étourdit" *The Letter*, 38.
16 "La mise en suspens de la signification dans la pratique de l'association libre révèle la question du sexe chez le parlant. Cette question ne trouve pas de réponse satisfaisante dans la réalité chromosomique ou anatomique. Le sexe chez le parlant n'est determine par aucun fond préalable au langage; il est absence de determination a priori." Christian Fierens, *Lecture de L'étourdit*, 55.
17 Jacques Lacan, "L'étourdit" *The Letter*, 46.
18 "[…] toutes les diverses fixations, les diverses modalités d'accès à la jouissance don't chacun dispose, qu'elles soient ou non conformes aux norms propres d'une époque." Colette Soler, *Ce que Lacan disait des femmes. Étude de psychanalyse* (Éditions du Champ lacanien, 2003), 211. For further details concerning the evolution of Lacan's teaching see the masterful reconstruction of Jacques-Alain Miller, "Les six paradigmes de la jouissance," *La Cause freudienne, Revue de Psychanalyse* 43 (1999).
19 Jacques Lacan, "L'étourdit" *The Letter*, 56.
20 "Et à prendre acte du reel, on en allège le poids, tout en mettant fin aux fausses espérences que génère le mirage de la vérité." Colette Soler, *Ce que Lacan disait des femmes*, 90.
21 "A partir du circuit impliqué par l'inconscient, se dégagent deux universels ('les deux sexes') qui séparent chez les parlants, non pas deux types d'être, non pas deux genres ou deux espèces, mais deux logiques ou, mieux, deux parties logiques indépendantes du sexe biologique." Christian Fierens, *Lecture de L'étourdit*, 93.

22 For a detailed explanation of the manner in which each of Lacan's formulas responds to those of *On Interpretation*, see Guy Le Gauffey, *Le Pastout de Lacan, Consistance logique, conséquences cliniques* (EPEL, 2006).

23 Jacques Lacan, *On Feminine Sexuality*, 78.

24 "C'est la politique du sujet contre la politique collectivisable du discours regnant. La politique de la psychanalyse a alors pour vocation de changer quelque peu l'économie de jouissance qui s'établit entre le sujet, objectuer à la jouissance universalisée, et le discours, administrateur de ladite jouissance." Javier Saez, *Théorie queer et psychanalyse*, 120.

25 Monique Wittig, "The Mark of Gender" in *The Straight Mind and Other* Essays (Beacon Press, 1992), 76.

26 "[...] elle semble encore trop fixée à son opposition au symbolique hétéronormatif, d'inspiration lévi-strausienne, figeant Lacan à l'époque de son 'retour à Freud' et de la complétude du symbolique, méconnaissant peut-être l'importance de la mutation opérée dans sa conceptualisation quand il donne de plus en plus de primauté au 'réel.'" Alain Lemosof, "Roc de *queer*" in *Sexualités, genres et mélancholie*, ed. by Monique David-Ménard (Campagne Première, 2009), 116. With this in mind, for Clotilde Leguil, Butler "says nothing about the real other than that it arises out of the manner in which the Lacanians speak" ("ne dit rien sur le reel si ce n'est qu'il est issu de a façon de parler des lacaniens") Clotilde Leguil, "Sur le genre des femmes selon Lacan" in *Subversion lacanienne des théroies du genre*, ed. by Fabian Fajnwaks and Clotilde Leguil (Editions Michèle, 2015), 60. In the same collection of esasys, Pierre-Gilles Guéguen affirms "We can say that *gender studies* have attempted to respond to the confusion of sex without wanting to know [...] what the unconscious held for each of the protesters. Without wanting to refer to the experience of the real in analysis and through analysis" ("Disons que les *gender studies* one tenté de répondre aux embarrass du sexe sans vouloir savoir [...] quel sort réservait l'inconscient à chacun des protestaires. Sans vouloir se référer à l'expérience du reel dans l'analyse et par l'analyse.") Pierre-Gilles Guéguen, "Le suppose troisième sexe" in *Subversion lacanienne des théroies du genre*, 136. For Marie Jejcic, "Butler decentres psychoanalysis from the real of the impossible sexual relation" ("Butler décentre la psychanalyse du reel de l'impossible rapport sexuel") Marie Jejcic, "Pour introduire à la lecture de Trouble dans le genre" *Sex and Gender. La revue Lacanienne* 4 (2007), 31. According to Javier Saez, "Butler's analysis of the real is based upon a substantialization of the real, confounding it with the 'referent,' that is, in attributing content to this non-discursive and 'impossible' register." ("L'analyse de Butler sur le reel se base sur une substantialisation du reel, en le confondant avec 'référent,' c'est-à-dire, en attribuant un contenu à ce register non discursive et 'impossible.') Javier Saez, *Théorie queer et psychanalyse*, 125. Fabian Fajnwaks also criticizes the lack of accounting for the real by *queer* theorists, notably by Marie-Hélène Sam Bourcier, in Fabian Fajnwaks, "Cultures *queer*: altérité et homosexualités" in *Elles ont choisi*, ed. by Stella Harrison (Editions Michèle, 2013), 105.

27 Regarding this point Éric Laurent offers a key contribution to the reading of the final teachings of Lacan. See Éric Laurent, *L'Envers de la biopolitique: une écriture pour la jouissance* (Navarin, 2016).

28 Given the shifting terrain of publications, this note does not propose to exhaustively detail the debate. It seems to me that the debate between Butler and Žižek begins in Savoj Žižek, *The Sublime Object of Ideology* (Verso, 1989) and in particular in chapter 2 and 5, to which Butler responds in "Arguing with the Real" in Judith Butler, *Bodies That Matter, On the Discursive Limits of 'Sex'*

(Routledge, 1993), 181–223. Žižek replies to Butler in Savoj Žižek, *The Ticklish Subject: The Absent Centre of Political Ontology* (Verso, 1999), in particular in chapters 5 and 6. The following year a dialogue in three voices between the political philosopher Eresto Laclau was published, Judith Butler, Eresto Laclau, and Savoj Žižek, *Contingency, Hegemony, Universality: Contemporary Dialogues on the Left* (Verso, 2000). This limited commentary cannot take the contribution of Laclau into account. Butler comments on the terms of this debate in several interviews, Judith Butler, "Gender as Performance. An Interview With Judith Butler," *Radical Philosophy* 67 (Summer 1994), 32–39, and Olson, Gary A., and Lynn Worsham, "Changing the Subject: Judith Butler's Politics of Radical Resignification," *JAC* 20, 4 (2000): 727–765. http://www.jstor.org/stable/20866363.

29 Žižek's reading is, in part, inspired by the orientation given by Jacques-Alain Miller regarding Lacan's corpus, without always following all of the subtleties therein. This invaluable work, which remains partially unpublished is available online: http://jonathanleroy.be/2020/12/orientation-lacanienne-jacques-alain-miller/. It is also available in numerous journals and in several translations.

30 Judith Butler, *Bodies That Matter*, ix.

31 For example, in France, Sylviane Agacinski has, with arms wide open, embraced this interrogation of the performative to such a degree that it risks leading her into error as concerns the interest of Butler's thought. See Sylviane Agacinski, *Femmes entre sexe et genre* (Seuil, 2012).

32 On this subject, one can only refer, once again, to the work of Wendy Brown, one of Butler's frequent partners in conversation, and who has shown that, in reality, neo-liberal rationality is not so much accompanied by a consumerist tolerance that would make the most of what it is presented with, than it is by a return to a neo-conservative rationality. See Wendy Brown, *Les Habits neufs de la politique Mondiale* (Les Prairies ordinaires, 2007). See also Wendy Brown, "American Nightmare: Neoliberalism, neoconservatism and De-Democratization," *Political Theory* 34, 6, (2006): 690–714.

33 Slavoj Žižek, "Class Struggle or Postmodernism? Yes, Please!" in Judith Butler, Eresto Laclau, and Savoj Žižek, *Contingency, Hegemony, Universality*, 98.

34 Slavoj Žižek, "Class Struggle or Postmodernism? Yes, Please!" in Judith Butler, Eresto Laclau, and Savoj Žižek, *Contingency, Hegemony, Universality*, 98.

35 Slavoj Žižek, "*Da Capo senza Fine*" in Judith Butler, Eresto Laclau, and Savoj Žižek, *Contingency, Hegemony, Universality*, 220.

36 This is precisely what the very interesting collection of texts and testimonies edited by Zena Sharman testifies to. See Zena Sharman (ed.), *The Remedy. Queer and Trans Voices on Health and Health Care* (Arsenal Pulp Press, 2016).

37 Slavoj Žižek, "Class Struggle or Postmodernism? Yes, Please!" in Judith Butler, Eresto Laclau, and Savoj Žižek, *Contingency, Hegemony, Universality*, 98.

38 Slavoj Žižek, "*Da Capo senza Fine*" in Judith Butler, Eresto Laclau, and Savoj Žižek, *Contingency, Hegemony, Universality*, 223.

39 For a definition of this term see Bernard Steigler, *The Decadence of Industrial Democracies: Disbelief and Discredit, Volume 1,* trans. Daniel Ross and Suzanne Arnold (Polity, 2011).

40 Judith Butler, *Giving an Account of Oneself* (Fordham University Press, 2005), 51.

41 While neither the imaginary nor the symbolic appear in Butler's text, her demonstration echoes, point for point, the critiques of Javier Saez in Javier Saez, *Théorie queer et psychanalyse*, 124. "Butler's insistence on the consubstantiality between the body and the ego illustrates her omission of one of the essential points of psychoanalysis, that which precisely affirms that desire springs forth

from the incommensurability between the body and the subject. For Lacan, there is a radical separation between the body and the subject, and between the subject and the object, which configures desire and the impossibility of its satisfaction. The subject finds itself separated from itself." / "L'insistance de Butler sur la consubstantialité entre le corps et l'ego montre son oubli d'un des points essentiels de la psychanalyse, laquelle affirme précisément que le désir surgit de l'incommensurabilité entre le corps et le sujet. Pour Lacan, il y a separation radicale entre le corps et le sujet, et entre le sujet et l'objet, ce qui configure le désir et l'impossibilité de sa satisfaction." *Giving an Account of Oneself* offers nothing more.

42 Judith Butler, *Giving an Account of Oneself*, 52.
43 Judith Butler, *Giving an Account of Oneself*, 53.
44 Judith Butler, *Giving an Account of Oneself*, 58.
45 Judith Butler, *Giving an Account of Oneself*, 54.
46 Jacques Lacan, "L'étourdit" *The Letter*, 56.
47 Sigmund Freud, "'A Child is Being Beaten': A Contribution to the Study of the Origin of Sexual Perversions" in *The Standard Edition of the Complete Psychological Works of Sigmund Freud*. Vol. XVII, 175–204.
48 Savoj Žižek, *The Ticklish Subject*, 271.
49 Savoj Žižek, *The Ticklish Subject*, 272.
50 Slavoj Žižek, "*Da Capo senza Fine*" in Judith Butler, Eresto Laclau, and Savoj Žižek, *Contingency, Hegemony, Universality*, 221.
51 Slavoj Žižek, "Class Struggle or Postmodernism? Yes, Please!" in Judith Butler, Eresto Laclau, and Savoj Žižek, *Contingency, Hegemony, Universality*, 110–111.
52 This is, in any case, the point of view of Tim Dean, "Lacan and Queer Theory," as well as of Javier Saez, *Théorie queer et psychanalyse* and Fabian Fajnwaks, "Cultures *queer*: Altérité et homosexualités."
53 Slavoj Žižek, "*Da Capo senza Fine*" in Judith Butler, Eresto Laclau, and Savoj Žižek, *Contingency, Hegemony, Universality*, 249.
54 Judith Butler, *Bodies That Matter*, 205.
55 Judith Butler, "Competing Universalities" in Judith Butler, Eresto Laclau, and Savoj Žižek, *Contingency, Hegemony, Universality*, 167.
56 Judith Butler, *Bodies That Matter*, 220–221.
57 Judith Butler, *Bodies That Matter*, 206.
58 Judith Butler, *Bodies That Matter*, 207.
59 Judith Butler, *Bodies That Matter*, 222.
60 Michel Foucault, "Maurice Blanchot: The Thought from Outside," *Foucoult Blanchot*, trans. Brian Massumi (Zone Books, 1987), 57.
61 Judith Butler, "Competing Universalities" in Judith Butler, Eresto Laclau, and Savoj Žižek, *Contingency, Hegemony, Universality*, 171.
62 Slavoj Žižek, "*Da Capo senza Fine*" in Judith Butler, Eresto Laclau, and Savoj Žižek, *Contingency, Hegemony, Universality*, 258–259.
63 See Jacques Lacan, *On the Names-of-the-Father*, trans. Bruce Fink (Polity, 2013). See also the excellent study of the logic of this subject given by Jacques-Alain Miller, "Petite introduction à *L'Au-dèla de l'oedipe,*" *La Cause freudienne* 21 (1992).
64 Anne Fausto-Sterling, *Sexing the Body. Gender Politics and the Construction of Sexuality* (Basic Books, 2000), 194.
65 Anne Fausto-Sterling, *Sexing the Body*, 3.
66 Jacques Lacan, *L'Identification. 1961–1962. Le séminaire, Livre IX*, unpublished. Lesson 30 May 1962. This particularly complex seminar is almost entirely articulated around the subject of topology so as to illustrate the

regression that underlies the analytic experience. Lacan also takes up the image of an ant as it wanders along a Möbius band to illustrate "a lack for which the symbol cannot compensate. This is not an absence that the symbol can counter." See Jacques Lacan, *Anxiety, The Seminar of Jacques Lacan. Book X 1962–1963*, ed. Jacques-Alain Miller, trans. A.R. Price (Polity, 2014), 136.
67 Anne Fausto-Sterling, *Sexing the Body*, 31.
68 Anne Fausto-Sterling, *Sexing the Body*, 253.
69 Jacques Lacan, *On Feminine Sexuality*, 67.
70 Anne Fausto-Sterling, *Sexing the Body*, 22.
71 Anne Fausto-Sterling, *Sexing the Body*, 42.
72 Anne Fausto-Sterling, *Sexing the Body*, 22.
73 Jacques Lacan, *On Feminine Sexuality*, 117.
74 Jacques Lacan, *On Feminine Sexuality*, 55.
75 Sigmund Freud, "A Difficulty in the Path of Psycho-analysis" in *The Standard Edition of the Complete Psychological Works of Sigmund Freud*. Vol. XVII, 143.
76 Jacques Lacan, *On Feminine Sexuality*, 79.
77 Jacques Lacan, *On Feminine Sexuality*, 87.
78 Jacques Lacan, *On Feminine Sexuality*, 92.
79 Jacques Lacan, "L'étourdit" *The Letter*, 34.
80 Jacques Lacan, *On Feminine Sexuality*, 93.
81 Jacques Lacan, *On Feminine Sexuality*, 93.
82 Concerning the antiphilosophy of Lacan, see Jorge Alemán, *L'Antifilosofia di Jacques Lacan* (Franco Angeli, 2003).
83 Jacques Lacan, *... or Worse, The Seminar of Jacques Lacan. Book XIX 1971–1972*, ed. Jacques Alain Miller, trans. A. R. Price (Polity, 2018), 92.
84 Jacques Lacan, *On Feminine Sexuality*, 76.
85 Jacques Lacan, *On Feminine Sexuality*, 80.
86 Sigmund Freud, "The Dissolution of the Oedipus Complex" in *The Standard Edition of the Complete Psychological Works of Sigmund Freud*. Vol. XIX, 178.
87 See, Anne Fausto-Sterling, "The Five Sexes" *The Sciences* 3 (1993): 20–25. See also Anne Fausto-Sterling, "The Five Sexes, Revisited" *The Sciences* 18 (2000): 18–23.
88 Anne Fausto-Sterling, *Sexing the Body*, 78.
89 Fausto-Sterling remarks that "success in gender assignment has traditionally been defined as living in that gender as a heterosexual." Anne Fausto-Sterling, "The Five Sexes, Revisited," 22.
90 Anne Fausto-Sterling, "The Five Sexes," 24.
91 Anne Fausto-Sterling, "The Five Sexes," 24.
92 Anne Fausto-Sterling, "The Five Sexes," 24.
93 "[…] recourir au pastout […] soit aux impasses de la logique." Jacques Lacan, "L'étourdit" in *Autres Écrits*, 479.
94 "[…] faire fixion autre du réel." Jacques Lacan, "L'étourdit" in *Autres Écrits*, 479.
95 "[…] l'impossible qui le fixe de la structure du langage. C'est aussi bien tracer la voie don't se retrouve en chaque discours e reel don't il s'enroule, et renvoyer les mythes don't il se supplée ordinairement." Jacques Lacan, "L'étourdit" in *Autres Écrits*, 479.
96 Jacques Lacan, "L'étourdit" in *Autres Écrits*, 491.
97 Eve Kosofsky Sedgwick, "Making Gay Meanings" in *The Weather in Proust* (Duke University Press, 2011), 188.
98 Eve Kosofsky Sedgwick, "Making Gay Meanings," 188.
99 Eve Kosofsky Sedgwick, "Making Gay Meanings," 188. [Author's italics]

100 Michel Foucault, *The Order of Things. An Archealogy of Human Sciences* (Vintage Books, 1994), 387.
101 Gilles Deleuze, *Difference and* Repetition, trans. Paul Patton (Columbia University Press, 1994), 107.

Bibliography

Agacinski, Sylviane. *Femmes entre sexe et genre*. Seuil, 2012.

Alemán, Jorge. *L'Antifilosofia di Jacques Lacan*. Franco Angeli, 2003.

Brown, Wendy. "American Nightmare: Neoliberalism, neoconservatism and De-Democratization." *Political Theory* 34, 6 (2006) : 690–714.

Brown, Wendy. *Les Habits neufs de la politique Mondiale*. Les Prairies ordinaires, 2007.

Butler, Judith. *Bodies That Matter, On the Discursive Limits of "Sex."*Routledge, 1993.

Butler, Judith. "Gender as Performance. An Interview With Judith Butler." *Radical Philosophy* 67 (Summer 1994): 32–39.

Butler, Judith. *Giving an Account of Oneself*. Fordham University Press, 2005.

Butler, Judith, Eresto Laclau, and Savoj Žižek. *Contingency, Hegemony, Universality: Contemporary Dialogues on the Left*. Verso, 2000.

Dean, Tim. "Lacan and Queer Theory" in *The Cambridge Companion to Lacan*. Edited by Jean-Michel Rabaté. Cambridge University Press, 2003: 238–252.

Deleuze, Gilles. *Difference and Repetition*. Translated by Paul Patton. Columbia University Press, 1994.

Fajnwaks, Fabian. "Cultures queer: Altérité et homosexualités." In *Elles ont choisi*. Edited by Stella Harrison. Editions Michèle, 2013.

Fausto-Sterling, Anne. "The Five Sexes" *The Sciences* 3 (1993): 20–25.

Fausto-Sterling, Anne. "The Five Sexes, Revisited" *The Sciences* 18 (2000): 18–23.

Fausto-Sterling, Anne. *Sexing the Body. Gender Politics and the Construction of Sexuality*. Basic Books, 2000.

Fierens, Christian. *Lecture de L'Étourdit. Lacan 1972*. L'Harmattan, 2002.

Foucault, Michel. "Maurice Blanchot: The Thought from Outside." In *Foucoult Blanchot*. Translated by Brian Massumi. Zone Books, 1987.

Foucault, Michel. *The Order of Things. An Archealogy of Human Sciences*. Vintage Books, 1994.

Freud, Sigmund. *The Standard Edition of the Complete Psychological Works of Sigmund Freud*. Edited by James Strachey, Anna Freud, and Angela Richards. Hogarth Press, 1953–1974.

Guéguen, Pierre-Gilles. "Le suppose troisième sexe." In *Subversion lacanienne des théroies du genre*. Edited by Fabian Fajnwaks and Clotilde Leguil. Editions Michèle, 2015.

Jejcic, Marie. "Pour introduire à la lecture de Trouble dans le genre." *Sex and Gender. La revue Lacanienne* 4 (2007).

Lacan, Jacques. *L'Identification. 1961–1962. Le séminaire, Livre* IX. Unpublished.

Lacan, Jacques. *The Four Fundamental Concepts of Psychoanalysis. The Seminar of Jacques Lacan. Book XI 1963–1964*. Edited by Jacques-Alain Miller. Translated by Alan Sheridan. W.W. Norton & Company, 1978.

Lacan, Jacques. *The Ethics of Psychoanalysis, The Seminar of Jacques Lacan. Book VII 1959–1960*. Edited by Jacques-Alain Miller. Translated by Dennis Porter. Routledge, 1992.

Lacan, Jacques. *On Feminine Sexuality, The Limits of Love and Knowledge, The Seminar of Jacques Lacan. Book XX*. Edited by Jacques-Alain Miller. Translated by Bruce Fink. W.W. Norton & Company, 1998.

Lacan, Jacques. *Autres Écrits*. Seuil, 2001.

Lacan, Jacques. "L'étourdit" Translated by Cormac Gallagher. *The Letter* 41. (2009): 31–80.

Lacan, Jacques. *On the Names-of-the-Father*. Translated by Bruce Fink. Polity, 2013.

Lacan, Jacques. *Anxiety, The Seminar of Jacques Lacan. Book X 1962–1963*. Edited by Jacques-Alain Miller. Translated by A.R. Price. Polity, 2014.

Lacan, Jacques. *... or Worse, The Seminar of Jacques Lacan. Book XIX 1971–1972*. Edited by Jacques-Alain Miller. Translated by A.R. Price. Polity, 2018.

Laurent, Éric. *L'Envers de la biopolitique: Une écriture pour la jouissance*. Navarin, 2016.

Le Gauffey, Guy. *Le Pastout de Lacan, Consistance logique, conséquences cliniques*. EPEL, 2006.

Leguil, Clotilde. "Sur le genre des femmes selon Lacan." In *Subversion lacanienne des théroies du genre*. Edited by Fabian Fajnwaks and Clotilde Leguil. Editions Michèle, 2015.

Lemosof, Alain. "Roc de *queer*." In *Sexualités, genres et mélancholie*. Edited by Monique David-Ménard. Campagne Première, 2009.

Melman, Charles "Édito," *Le Bulletin Lacanien 4: "Sex and gender"*. Association Lacanienne internationale, 2008.

Miller, Jacques-Alain. "Petite introduction à *L'Au-dèla de l'oedipe*," *La Cause freudienne, Revue de Psychanalyse* 21 (1992).

Miller, Jacques-Alain. "Les six paradigmes de la jouissance," *La Cause freudienne, Revue de Psychanalyse* 43 (1999).

Olson, Gary A., and Lynn Worsham. "Changing the Subject: Judith Butler's Politics of Radical Resignification." *JAC* 20, 4 (2000): 727–765. http://www.jstor.org/stable/20866363.

Saez, Javier. *Théorie queer et psychanalyse*. EPEL, 2005.

Sedgwick, Eve Kosofsky. "Making Gay Meanings." In *The Weather in Proust*. Duke University Press, 2011, 183–189.

Sharman, Zena (ed.). *The Remedy. Queer and Trans Voices on Health and Health Care*. Arsenal Pulp Press, 2016.

Soler, Colette. *Ce que Lacan disait des femmes. Étude de psychanalyse*. Éditions du Champ lacanien, 2003.

Steigler, Bernard. *The Decadence of Industrial Democracies: Disbelief and Discredit*, Volume 1. Translated by Daniel Ross and Suzanne Arnold. Polity, 2011.

Wittig, Monique. *The Straight Mind and Other Essays*. Beacon Press, 1992.

Žižek, Savoj. *The Sublime Object of Ideology*. Verso, 1989.

Žižek, Savoj. *The Ticklish Subject: The Absent Centre of Political Ontology*. Verso, 1999.

Conclusion

What did I want to write to my friends? That I am a "faggot"? Do they not know this already? Have I not already filled their ears to the brim with my coming out? That society is stuffed full of prejudices? That education, the media, smutty discourse and well-meaning morality alike all conspire to perpetuate the heterosexual norm? Most of them are not ignorant of this, and each and every one, in their own manner, force themselves to adopt the attitudes necessary to avoid clichés and to have a little more consideration for differences. That their clinical practice no longer needed to operate through the framework of the Oedipal in order to hear and understand the life stories that are shelled out within their rooms? Have they not, in all this time, already gained insight into hearing the complaints of those who have grown up in reconstructed, mono-parental, postmodern families? That *the* difference between the sexes has, for the longest time, been an excuse behind which the inequalities of the patriarchy have been hidden, and that one has had to put the weight of this into perspective? On this last point, perplexed, certain among them continue to consider that it is all very well to invoke anatomical exceptions and the most fantastic cultural constructions, but that the world despite all rhetoric artifice, always ends up dividing itself along the lines of this opposition between masculine and feminine…

What did I want to write to my friends? That I was a psychoanalyst. They no longer care about that and haven't for ages. That my silence was not indicative of my judgement? Were they not so preoccupied in sounding forth their own claims and demands that they didn't pay the least bit of attention? That their suffering and their lives merit every bit as much attention as that which is paid to others? Is this not precisely the point of their struggles? Were they to triumph in this regard, would their souls find peace? They would like to find out. That deconstructing knowledge and practices, that taking responsibility for one's gestures and body, that demanding the recognition of one's pleasure does not deliver one from the unconscious? Perhaps, but they all have so much more to do before their consciousnesses are liberated…

DOI: 10.4324/9781003612735-6

In too clearly wanting to assemble each and every one, in shaking up the critiques of some and the discontent of others, in moving from one side to the other, in too forcefully pressing one *against* the other, in shifting from one foot to the other, in swinging from one position to the other, has my writing and my tumultuous embraces had no other effect than to, in the final account, attract new enemies? In the end, does the vigorous embrace between the *queer* critiques and the practice of psychoanalysis not lead us to rekindle the dissatisfaction of one and of all? At times I may have drawn a less than flattering portrait of lady psychoanalysis. I may have caricatured her tired features, her taciturn complexion, her Pythian allure of sibyllic flights of fancy. At others I may have poured cold water on the flames of revolution. I may have blunted the strategies of resistance so as to renew the instruments of oppression. On both sides I stumbled and tripped, offside and transgressive.

These pages have tried to enact an exhausting contortion: maintain the corrosive energy of the unconscious *and* of the *queer*, restore the image of the equivocal *and* sing to the glory of the performative, touch the intimate *and* the most singular in order to shift norms *and* politics. Ethics is an exhausting sport: we beef up our contradictions, we withstand tension, we push our flexibility to the limit. I have taken the gamble of an inexhaustible *queer* rage and the eternal youth of the unconscious. I have bet on the force of militancy *and* of desire to renew the tonalities of the psychoanalytic process. Without a doubt, certain subjectivities are able to waltz in harmony with the thrum of a major key. Light as a feather, they move in the step and rhythm of a dated venetian dance. But these chamber dances do not suit everyone. It seemed necessary to me to extend out the theory and the clinic so as to accommodate the ballet of minor people. Their choreography ceaselessly reinvents itself in the steps and along the stops of the cure. Some may have found their gymnastics to be needless. Others may complain about their postures. None will be saved from this fatigue.

May my friends forgive me: "if friendship calls upon the community through writing, it can only except itself (friendship for the exigency of writing which excludes all friendship)."[1] The link that I have tried to weave between *queer* theory and psychoanalysis was orientated by the interest of directing our sight Outside: "as that which prevents, precedes, and dissolves the possibility of any personal relation."[2] Unattainable horizon. Positioned *in between* both ambitious and incommode. Such a journey momentarily condemns one to exile, to wandering or to solitude. It provokes a crisis in the well-worn paths in order to discover a passion renewed, intensities rekindled, and colours hitherto unseen. These are the indispensable conditions required to reaffirm a communal task that is without end.

I believe that the voices and the paths of desire have reached a courageous breathlessness. Panting, we set off, session after session, in an "affective Athleticism," "an athleticism of becoming that reveals only forces that are not its own."[3] Therein lies a search for a precarious balance, between contradictions, frictions, and contempt. Hold the discomfort close. Maintain an uncomfortable balancing act. Aim for a true escape from *being*. Await the *and*: Lacanian *and* Deleuzian *and queer and* postfeminist *and* post-Oedipean *and…*

Become the unconscious in a minor key.

Notes

1 Maurice Blanchot, *The Unavowable Community*, trans. Pierre Joris (Station Hill, 1988), 24.
2 Maurice Blanchot, "The Essential Solitude" in *The Space of Literature*, trans. Anne Smock (University of Nebraska Press, 1982), 31.
3 Gilles Deleuze and Félix Guattari, *What is Philosophy?* trans. Hugh Tomlinson and Graham Burchell (Columbia University Press, 1994), 172.

Bibliography

Blanchot, Maurice. "The Essential Solitude." In *The Space of Literature*. Translated by Anne Smock. University of Nebraska Press, 1982.

Blanchot, Maurice. *The Unavowable Community*. Translated by Pierre Joris. Station Hill, 1988.

Gilles Deleuze and Félix Guattari, *What is Philosophy?* Translated by Hugh Tomlinson and Graham Burchell. Columbia University Press, 1994.

Index

For Product Safety Concerns and Information please contact our
EU representative GPSR@taylorandfrancis.com Taylor & Francis
Verlag GmbH, Kaufingerstraße 24, 80331 München, Germany